DISCOURSE ANALYSIS AND APPLICATIONS
Studies in Adult Clinical Populations

DISCOURSE ANALYSIS AND APPLICATIONS
Studies in Adult Clinical Populations

Edited By
Ronald L. Bloom
Hofstra University
Loraine K. Obler
City University of New York
Susan De Santi
New York University Medical Center
Jonathan S. Ehrlich
Private Practice, Edison, New Jersey

Psychology Press
Taylor & Francis Group
NEW YORK AND HOVE

First published by Lawrence Erlbaum Associates, Inc., Publishers

This edition published 2013 by Psychology Press

Psychology Press	Psychology Press
711 Third Avenue	27 Church Road
New York	Hove
NY 10017	East Sussex, BN3 2FA

First issued in paperback 2014

Psychology Press is an imprint of the Taylor & Francis Group, an informa business

Cover design by Rosalind Orland

Library of Congress Cataloging-in-Publication Data

Discourse analysis and applications : studies in adult clinical populations / edited by Ronald L. Bloom . . . [et al.].
p. cm.
Includes bibliographical references and index.
ISBN 0-8058-1365-9 (cloth : acid-free paper)
1. Brain damage—Patients—Language. 2. Discourse analysis.
I. Bloom, Ronald L.
RC423.D56 1994
616.85'5—dc20 94-665
CIP

ISBN 13: 978-1-138-87640-8 (pbk)
ISBN 13: 978-0-8058-1365-4 (hbk)

To *Deborah* and *Jessica*—R.L.B.

To *Nathaniel*—L.K.O.

To *Mary* and *David*—S.D.

To *Rachel*, *Joshua*, and *Yosefa*—J.E.

Contents

Preface

For more than a century, brain-damaged adults have been examined to reveal information about how language is organized in the brain. Studies of adults with left-brain damage have led to certain widely accepted neuroanatomic correlates between lesion site and impaired linguistic behavior. Historically, models of brain and language behavior have been constructed primarily on the basis of comprehension and production of words and sentences in patients with damage to the dominant hemisphere. Within recent decades, linguistic analysis has expanded beyond word and sentence-level evaluation to include analysis of discourse. The basic premise of discourse analysis is that meanings are conveyed through extended units of language where participants attempt to share perspectives and exchange knowledge about the world, not by words and sentences alone.

Systematic examination of discourse provides a rich source of data for describing the complex relationships among language, social context, and the cognitive processes that underlie discourse comprehension and production. When studied across different clinical populations, discourse analysis provides an optimal opportunity for developing dynamic models of brain and language that more fully account for the complexity of language use in social contexts. Accordingly, studies presented in this volume have a dual focus, namely, to examine the implications of discourse research on neurolinguistic theories and to evaluate the contribution of discourse analysis to understanding the clinical status of patients with brain damage.

The chapters in this volume report patterns of preserved and impaired discourse behavior in normal adults and in different adult clinical populations. Various discourse types or genres, each with its own internal structure, are discussed. Conversational, narrative, procedural, expository, and instructional discourse genres may be distinguished from each other by the roles and expectations speakers and listeners form during communication. Conversational discourse is a dialogue that involves the speaker and listener in an interactive exchange of information. By contrast, narrative discourse is a monologue where a speaker describes a sequence of real or imagined events to a relatively nonverbal listener. Narratives are composed of a setting (i.e., the characters and story context) and one or more episodes (i.e., the events, responses, and consequences of the story) that may be interrelated. Procedural discourse directs a listener how to do something in a series of chronological or conceptually related steps, whereas expository discourse embellishes on a general topic in no particular sequence. Instructional discourse involves the specific style of communication that takes place between a teacher and student. Specific to each discourse genre are social roles and expectations that are negotiated and conveyed in a rule-governed, predictable manner.

Contributors to this volume describe numerous tasks designed to elicit a variety of discourse genres. Elicitation methods vary in terms of the stimuli or stimulus types used and the cognitive demands of each task. For example, narratives elicited by stimulus pictures permit the investigator to control for the content and complexity of the information that is expressed. Story-recall tasks also permit the investigator to load the story with particular types of content while challenging the short-term memory of the speaker. Elicitation style may affect conversational discourse. Certainly, the relevance of the topic to the speaker can influence the quantity and quality of language produced. Topic selection also influences what the speaker may assume about the knowledge level of the listener. Degree of familiarity between communication partners may affect the selection of referents that are discussed and the linguistic options used to encode reference.

Discourse analysis includes a host of techniques designed to describe how subjects order information and relate ideas across sentences. Numerous abstract units and linguistic devices have been targeted in order to examine those aspects of discourse that govern cohesion, organization, and topic manipulation. In terms of discourse production, narrative, expository, and procedural genres have two broad levels of analysis. Macrostructure analysis examines the global organization of the essential and optional elements of discourse. Such an analysis evaluates a speaker's ability to impart the central idea of the story and to synthesize its essence by stating the moral or recounting the gist. Microstructure analysis evaluates how the use of specific linguistic devices affect the cohesion or the semantic relations that bind linguistic items together across sentences. Microstructure analysis may examine, for example, speakers' use of reference or their ability to conjoin phrases and sentences through the use of conjunctions. In addition to these levels of analysis, conversational discourse introduces the opportunity to examine the turn-taking behavior of communication partners as well as breakdowns in conversation and the strategies employed to repair breakdowns. Because of the role expectations inherent in instructional discourse, the manner in which social position is verbally negotiated may be evaluated in this discourse genre. In terms of comprehension, coherence (i.e., how the listener interprets the sense of the message) may be examined. Although the methods of analysis and the abstract units of study that are presented in this book vary, virtually all of the studies view language as a dynamic social process shared by a listener and speaker.

GOALS OF THE BOOK

One major goal of this book is to examine current theoretical issues concerning models of discourse processing via study of their breakdown resulting from damage to the central nervous system. For example, to increase understanding of the issues surrounding brain laterality and localization, studies that examine discourse following a focal lesion to either the left or right hemisphere are described. The second major goal is to investigate what discourse analysis contributes to our understanding of the linguistic, cognitive, and social aspects of disorder in different clinical populations. In addition to examining patients with focal brain damage, studies of the discourse of adults with Alzheimer's disease, closed head injury, learning disability, and mental retardation are presented. The third major goal of this book is to explore the clinical utility of discourse analysis in different adult populations. The authors provide evidence that examining discourse increases understanding of the linguistic, social, and cognitive consequences of the particular disorder under investigation and that it does so in ways that suggest new avenues for rehabilitation. The fourth goal is to provide readers with a broad range of methodological approaches to evaluate discourse in adults. The studies presented in this volume highlight the potential of discourse analysis for differentiating among various language disorders and for capturing aspects of communication breakdown in individual patients.

PLAN OF THE BOOK

This volume contains an introduction and 12 chapters organized to provide an appreciation of analytic discourse techniques and applications. In the introductory chapter, Duchan examines some of the broader theoretical issues involved in the study of discourse through an exploration of the historical roots and evolution of analytic techniques. In order to look at discourse parameters of brain-damaged patients, data on the range of discourse behavior from normals of similar ages is required. In chapter 2, Obler, Au, Kugler, Tocco, Melvold, and Albert focus on issues that arise when describing regularities and variations that exist in the discourse of healthy elderly adults. This chapter summarizes narrative data from three age groups of men and women: 30-year-olds, 50-year-olds, and 70-year-olds.

Narratives were examined for content units, links between these units, grammatical categories, use of indefinite terms, extra-story comments, and paragrammatisms.

Chapter 3, written by Ulatowska and Chapman, presents a neurolinguistic framework for categorizing discourse performance in left-brain-damaged aphasic patients. The authors report that although the macrostructure of discourse is relatively intact following aphasia, there is a disruption to information structure on tasks that require story content to be condensed or generalized. Use of conversational discourse genre to improve communication in certain aphasic patients is discussed.

Haravon, Obler, and Sarno (chapter 4) present a systematic approach for the microanalysis of discourse. This chapter details a methodology for coding samples of discourse. Examples of clear-cut analyses are given, as well as instances where analysis is challenging. The techniques presented should be useful in language assessment, designing treatment, and monitoring subtle linguistic changes that occur in the course of recovery.

In chapter 5, Bloom reviews research that has examined discourse in patients with unilateral left- or right-brain damage. Theories about hemispheric responsibility and discourse production are discussed. Based on the description of spared and impaired language skills that emerge in both patient groups, a preliminary model of discourse production is proposed. Clinical applications for working with aphasic and right hemisphere-damaged patients are discussed.

Conversational discourse of closed head injured adults is discussed by Coelho, Liles, and Duffy in chapter 6. Two studies that illustrate the clinical utility of assessing communicative abilities of these patients in natural contexts are summarized. In the first study, analytic measures of intersentential cohesion and episode structure were applied to narratives collected longitudinally from closed head injured subjects. In the second study, conversational discourse of closed head injured patients is compared with that of aphasic subjects and normal controls. This chapter argues that the communication problems that emerge following closed head injury result directly from an impairment in language use.

In chapter 7, Domingo takes a close look at the instructional interactions of teachers and mentally retarded adults in a day treatment program. Examination of the pragmatic intentions expressed revealed that adults with mild to moderate mental retardation demonstrate the potential for self-regulation in dyadic interactions.

Oral story production in learning disabled adults is the focus of chapter 8. Roth and Spekman provide evidence of the relationship between narrative discourse proficiency and academic achievement. Narrative proficiency in this population is viewed from a developmental perspective, where certain difficulties are resolved by early adolescence and others persist into adulthood.

Chapters 9, 10, 11, 12, and 13 examine the ways discourse breaks down in Alzheimer's dementia. Ehrlich (chapter 9) reviews recent research in discourse production in patients with dementia of Alzheimer's type. Methodological problems are identified and suggestions for future research are provided. In chapter 10, Garcia and Joanette demonstrate how the conversational topic-shifting styles of patients with dementia may be operationalized.

Hamilton (chapter 11) examines the difficulty investigators have in differentiating between production and comprehension problems in the discourse of Alzheimer's patients. A single subject's requests for clarification are examined as they occurred in conversations with the examiner. Hamilton proposes that the problems underlying discourse in demented patients is a byproduct of an analytic approach that places responsibility for interpreting what is said in the researcher's hands.

De Santi, Koenig, Obler, and Goldberg (chapter 12) discuss methods employed to examine the cohesive devices used by patients with Alzheimer's disease and normal controls during conversational discourse. A series of increasingly more refined analyses directed at examining semantic and syntactic cohesive devices is presented.

In chapter 13, Causino Lamar, Obler, Knoefel, and Albert describe the communication of institutionalized patients with end-stage Alzheimer's disease. Two qualitatively distinct subgroups of patients emerged, identifiable through a hierarchy of relatively spared to severely impaired pragmatic behaviors. Strategies are proposed that may lead to improved conversation with these patients.

In summary, *Discourse Analysis and Applications: Studies in Adult Clinical Populations* presents both theoretical and clinical chapters that examine a variety of communication pathologies. Rather than endorsing a single approach to discourse elicitation or analysis, this volume provides a wide range of methodological approaches used to capture the features of language that give communication its content, shape, and texture. Although the spirit of this volume is exploratory, the outcome has been useful in introducing some functional and innovative analytic techniques and theories. Clinicians often report dissatisfaction with formal test batteries in that results are often at variance with clinical observation of performance in real-life situations. The methods proposed for examining discourse move the examiner closer to naturalistic sampling. The work in this volume suggests that discourse analysis provides clinically significant information that contributes to the understanding of the cognitive, linguistic, and social status of people with communication disorders. These studies provide the theoretical framework to support continuously evolving diagnostic and treatment paradigms for adults with communication pathologies.

Ronald L. Bloom

Chapter 1

Approaches to the Study of Discourse in the Social Sciences

Judith Duchan
State University of New York at Buffalo

Even though studies of discourse began in ancient times (e.g., Aristotle's *Poetics*), they have only recently come to the fore in the social sciences. Discourse studies are now becoming commonplace in anthropology (e.g., Clifford, 1988), history (e.g., White, 1981), sociology (e.g., Drew & Heritage, 1992), linguistics (e.g., Chafe, 1980; Halliday & Hasan, 1976), computer science (e.g., Frederiksen, Bracewell, Breuleux, & Renauld, 1990), psychology (e.g., van Dijk & Kintsch, 1983), education (Cazden, 1988), and neurolinguistics (Joanette & Brownell, 1990, as well as this volume). The stunning growth in the number of researchers studying discourse and in the number of studies published in the area is evidenced by the emergence in the social sciences of new journals (e.g., *Discourse Processes*, *Journal of Narrative and Life History*, *Text*), conferences on the topic, and books such as this dedicated solely to aspects of discourse.

The emphases of these relatively new research efforts differ from one another, depending on the discipline and the specific philosophy and goals of the researchers carrying them out. However varied, the studies together have the potential of dramatically changing what went before. Their effect on former thinking in the disciplines has yet to be realized. Some foresee a paradigm shift that will shake disciplinary grounds and require new looks at old truths (Gee, 1992). Others treat the new studies as a natural outgrowth of previous work following the natural progressions in their home discipline (Bloom, chapter 5, this volume; Halliday & Hasan, 1976).

The authors of the studies in this volume follow their sciences' natural progression in that they have used analyses that are logical extensions of what has been done before. The authors provide us with a coherent and specific approach to the study of discourse using well worked out methods to investigate new phenomena. That approach is linguistic in that it treats discourse as consisting of language constituents. Discourse is seen as ways in which sentences are combined to form meaningful wholes. The analyses in the studies are structural because they are aimed at uncovering the underlying structures around which the elements of the discourse corpus is organized. The studies are comparative in that the organizational structure of discourse produced by adults with disabilities is compared with that produced by adults without disabilities.

Although the studies all fall within the philosophy and methodology of a linguistic structuralist tradition, they differ considerably from one another in what they study and how they carry out their analyses. Studies are of different discourse genres, for example, with some examining their subjects' picture descriptions, others using storytelling and recall, and still others using instructional discourse. The elements studied within the genres also differ for the different research projects. Some researchers study small, micro-, or nearby relations between elements in the text such as local level cohesion devices (Coelho, Liles, & Duffy, chapter 6, this volume; and DeSanti, Koenig, Obler, & Goldberger, chapter 12, this volume); others focus on structures that affect more of the discourse—global or macrostructures such as themes, episodes, or morals (Coelho et al., chapter 6, this volume; Ulatowska, Chapman, & Johnson, chapter 3, this volume).

The studies in this book fit neatly with what is currently going on in the social sciences in the area of discourse studies. In this chapter I review and characterize the various ways researchers in the social sciences have been studying discourse in recent years in an effort to show the historical roots of the approaches taken by those in this book and to place the work in its context. I then present an overview of the literature on linguistic analyses of discourse. Finally, I suggest some future directions for research of this type, so as to be in keeping with this book's spirit of adventure and with its aim to pave new ways for studying those with communicative disorders.

APPROACHES TO DISCOURSE

The Thought Behind the Discourse. A strong impetus for studying discourse has been from the developments in "schema theory" in psychology and computer science (Mandler, 1984; Schank & Abelson, 1977). The theory holds that discourse is created, understood, and remembered in accordance with complex mental representations or conceptual schemas. (See Bartlett, 1932, for an earlier and well-developed rendition of this view as it applies to memory.) For example, a story that is structured like a fable will have a setting, a middle episode or episodes, and an ending. To know and expect this structure when dealing with a new or a familiar story is to have a schema about the structure of stories of this type (Mandler &

Johnson, 1977; Rumelhart, 1975; Stein & Glenn, 1979). Individuals who know the abstract structure of such stories use that knowledge whenever dealing with a particular story having such a format. Examples of schemata that have been hypothesized as structures underlying different types of discourse are *event scripts* used in creating and understanding event descriptions (Nelson, 1986), *story grammars* used in interpreting and recalling simple stories (Roth & Spekman, chapter 8, this volume; Stein & Glenn, 1979), and exchange structures governing the turn-taking etiquette of parties engaged in a classroom lesson, for example (Mehan, 1979).

The Creative Translation of Thought Into Language. The researchers who study the conceptual or schematic underpinnings of discourse have been critiqued for paying insufficient attention to how the schemas get translated into language. Bamberg (1991, p. 158), for example, criticized those who seem to be treating discourse as a direct mapping of language onto conceptual structures. He advocated a more complex view that regards the relationship between thoughts and their telling as being a highly creative one. Under the mapping view, stories should have the same time structure and subjective perspective as the experience being told about. The creative view presumes that the verbal expression of an experience involves many choices and is likely to differ from the original experience not only in its temporality but also in the personal point of view. Tellers, in order to make their tale more suspenseful and understandable, can highlight certain aspects of the event, alter temporal sequences, and shift perspectives to portray the feelings of other participants. Those with well-developed discourse competence will be able to choose a level of detail within which to cast their ideas. They can report what happened in outline form, as did the annalists of medieval times who listed events that occurred without ascribing motivation or a connection between them (White, 1981); they can create a more detailed depiction including motivation and connectivity to entertain an audience (Brewer & Lichtenstein, 1982), or they can provide excruciating detail such as that needed when producing descriptions as evidence in courtroom proceedings (Barry, 1991).

Discourse as Interpreted Text. Compatible with the creative view of discourse is the open text view that sees the language of the discourse as a skeletal rendition of its intended interpretation. A painted scene, even one that is a realistic version of the original scene, is only suggestive of the original. The painter as well as the viewer knows more about the painting than is shown directly: They must provide a third dimension to a two-dimensional surface, they must ascribe emotional content using the choice of colors and shapes, and they must relate the lines to the imagined scene in order to interpret them as horizons, trees, or mountains. Finally, they may want to evaluate the effort as a work of art, drawing on their previous experiences with the particular genre and knowledge of the work of other artists engaged in it. Similarly, someone describing a scene is also forced to create a skeletal version of the real or imagined scene, relying on the interpreter to read between the lines in order to arrive at the coherent and elaborated picture.

Not all discourse analysts subscribe to the open text view. Instead, they adopt a more closed text view and, for example, focus on the language of the text rather than on how authors and recipients interpret the text. Halliday and Hasan (1976) took a closed view of textual cohesion when they depicted textual elements as related, rather than regarding the interpreter of the text as the one who infers the relationship. In a closed text view anaphoric pronouns are described as getting their meaning through ties to earlier referring expressions in the text (Halliday & Hasan, 1976; Liles, 1985), rather than as being interpreted in accordance with focused elements in a mental representation.

Voice and Value Orientation as Expressed in Discourse. Various authors have studied emotionally laden aspects of discourse, or what Bamberg (1991) called the "value orientations" in the discourse. He included in this approach researchers who have studied the type and use of evaluative comments in narratives (e.g., Bamberg & Damrad-Frye, 1991; Labov & Waletsky, 1967; Reilly, 1992) as well as those who have studied the "voice" in which a segment of discourse is expressed (Bakhtin, 1985; Bamberg, 1991; Budwig, 1991, cited in Bamberg, 1991). Also within the value orientation approaches is the research that analyzes discourse describing emotionally laden experiences (Haviland & Goldston, in press; Hudson, Gebelt, Haviland, & Bentivenga, 1992). Finally, there are studies that compare discourse and communicative competence for discourse contexts that require emotionally laden expressions with those that do not (R. Bloom, Borod, Obler, & Gerstman, 1992; Hudson et al., 1992).

The Influences of Audience on an Author's Discourse Structuring. A number of research projects have investigated ways discourse is designed to fit the intended audience. Linguistic devices have been identified that signal a listener or reader about how to understand the narratives. Intensity markers such as "really" tell the audience what is important (Labov, 1984); words and phrases such as "so," "then," "anyway," "by the way" can be used to mark degree of continuity or discontinuity in the discourse (Duchan, Waltzman, & Meth, 1992; Schiffrin, 1987; Young, 1987), and syntactic and morphological and vocal indicators of subordination can be used to distinguish foreground from background information (Hopper, 1979). Authors as young as 4 years have been found to structure their discourse differently depending on whether their audience is presumed to be knowledgable or naive about the subject matter (Shatz & Gelman, 1973).

Discourse Expressions of Authority and Power. Discourse analyses have also been aimed at discovering the power relationships expressed between the writer or speaker and the audience. Noteworthy contributors to this approach are ethnographers whose own research reports have been the object of their discourse analyses. The conclusion from their analyses has been that the researchers typically take an authoritarian stance casting their subjects as subordinate "others" (Clifford, 1983; Geertz, 1988; Young, 1991).

Other researchers have examined the discourse for evidence of power relations between the subjects they are studying (e.g., Bedrosian & Prutting, 1978; Domingo, chapter 7, this volume). These authors have analyzed conversational bids, such as direct and indirect requests, as manifestations of underlying dominance relations among participants. They found a difference in requesting between dominant and submissive partners and that these expressions of dominance and submission differed with different contexts.

Discourse as Interaction. The emphases just described have had their focus on the author and textual contributions to the discourse structuring. There is also a healthy research literature that sees discourse as a two- or multiparty endeavor. Some studies show the influence of listeners' actions to the speakers' subsequent discourse production (e.g., Goodwin, 1981). Others, such as those who adopt the tenets of postmodernism, take the perspective of the audience as their point of departure, examining the readers' interpretation of texts (Rosenau, 1992). Still others examine the reciprocal contribution of both partners in the creation of a segment of discourse (Higginbotham, 1989).

The Functions of Discourse. Discourse has been subdivided into different genres based on the different functions served. Bruner (1986) took a global look at discourse function, looking at the functional differences in discourse genres. He viewed "argument" and "narrative" as having different functions in that "arguments convince one of their truth, stories of their lifelikeness" (p. 11). Conversational analysts study ways partners negotiate turn-taking during their conversational interactions. They also study in detail more circumscribed functions carried out sporadically such as that involved in the repairing of conversational breakdowns (Schegloff, Jefferson, & Sacks, 1977), issuing invitations (Drew, 1984), and delivering bad news during clinical interactions (Maynard, 1992). Finally, discourse functions have been found to be sensitive to cultural difference and thus to create difficulty in contexts of cultural mismatches (Heath, 1983; Michaels, 1981).

Discourse of Situations. Some researchers have confined their study of discourse to situated talk. They have, for example, examined the discourse requirements of various speech events such as lessons of the classroom (Cazden, 1988; Mehan, 1979), therapeutic interactions (Labov & Fanshel, 1977), or courtroom testimony (Barry, 1991). The findings indicate that events play a strong role in dictating or influencing the discourse structure, and that analysts of one type of discourse may not be able to generalize their findings to other discourse genres.

Modality Comparisons Between Oral and Written Discourse. There has been a group of important studies that has differentiated oral from written discourse, arguing that written discourse is not simply oral language written down (Chafe, 1985; Tannen, 1985; Westby, 1985). Rather, the modality differences, like event differences, influence the discourse. Even at the surface level of analysis one can differentiate oral from written discourse. A speaker engaging in oral face-to-face conversation can call on intonation, silences, gaze, postural, and gestural indicators to signal meaning. Writers, on the other hand, have at their disposal the use of linguistic devices of punctuation, paragraph indicators, lines, and headings (Tannen, 1985). At a deeper level, researchers have pointed to differences in syntax and types of coherence expressed by oral versus written discourse (Chafe, 1985; Westby, 1985).

Discourse Structure and Coherence. Discourse analysts have distinguished discourse coherence from discourse cohesion, with coherence having to do with the meaning assigned to the text and the cohesion with the way the text is structurally integrated. (See later for a discussion of cohesion.) Various authors who have studied discourse coherence have listed how content from different parts of the text can relate to one another. Hobbs (1990) identified occasion relations as ones in which one event, say a train arriving in Chicago, sets up an occasion in which a subsequent event takes place, the president gives a speech. Other coherence relations described by Hobbs are: evaluation relations (relating an element and its goal), ground-figure relations (relating an element to the listeners' prior knowledge), and expansion relations (moving between specific and general assertions).

Analysts studying coherence have developed ways of uncovering the causal structuring of event descriptions by examining what have been called *event chains* expressed within a plan or as part of an integrated series of activities (Kemper & Edwards, 1986; Trabasso, Secco, & van den Broek, 1984). Event descriptions as well as story plots typically include a depiction of states and actions that are caused or themselves cause other events. The nature of causality may be related to the aims of the participants in the story as is the case for actions carried out by a character. The character's motivation to achieve a goal and the specification of that goal ties conceptually to the actions the character engages in to achieve that goal. Causal chains can also be physical in origin as when conditions enable actions to take place or when actions are blocked by unexpected circumstances.

Processing Factors. Processing of discourse has been investigated by studying subjects' abilities to deal with discourse segments under various experimental manipulations. For example, comparisons have been made of subjects' abilities to recall discourse after different time intervals (Bartlett, 1932). A second way in which processing has been studied is to examine the way the discourse is delivered. For example, Obler, Au, Kugler, Melvold, Tocco, and Albert (chapter 2, this volume) studied voluminousness, Crago and Eriks-Brophy

(1994) studied the cross-cultural use of silence in discourse production, Marshall (1977) discussed problems in starting up and stopping, Haravon, Obler, and Sarno (chapter 4, this volume) examined occasions when subjects stop talking in midsentence, and Obler et al. (chapter 2, this volume) studied their subjects' use of *fillers* such as "um."

Clinical Approaches to Discourse. What makes this book unusual is its attention to the discourse of individuals who comprise different clinical groups. The approach is a normative one in that the discourse of subject groups is compared with that of age-matched subjects with no disability. The approach is also usually quantitative where the experimental and control groups are compared on the incidence of occurrence of an identified discourse structure. Among the comparisons are: number of initiations (Coelho et al., chapter 6, this volume); number of ambiguous referring expressions (Liles, 1985; Bloom, chapter 5, this volume), or number of times expected structural elements are absent (Roth & Spekman, chapter 8, this volume).

LINGUISTIC APPROACHES

The linguistic approach to the study of discourse is one in which the language of the text becomes the focus for examination. A common enterprise when taking a discourse perspective toward language structure is to identify structures in the language that signal information about how the discourse is organized. Constituents that are treated at the sentence-level of analysis, such as noun phrases, connectives, and verb phrases, are reexamined for their functions at the level of discourse. Noun phrases can be studied for their role in participant tracking (Grimes, 1975), connectives for their use in creating discourse cohesion (Duchan, Meth, & Waltzman, 1992; Halliday & Hasan, 1976; Coelho, Liles, & Duffey, chapter 6, this volume; Schiffrin, 1987), and aspects of the verb system can serve to mark temporality including shifts to a new discourse time (Almeida, in press).

Among the discourse jobs that the language needs to do are (a) referencing and tracking the participants; (b) marking the nature relationships between adjacent sentences (local level cohesion indicators); (c) marking the relationships between larger units of discourse such as episodes (global level indicators); (d) tracking the spatial, temporal, and personal perspectives on the discourse (deictic elements); (e) indicating plans, motivation, and causation; and (f) indicating genre framing shifts such as moves from conversations to stories.

Referencing and Tracking the Participants. In order to make discourse understandable and to help an audience keep track of the elements being referred to, an author must at first identify those elements and, once they are focused on, must help the listener or reader keep track of which ones are being referred to. Noun phrases are the constituents of the language that do most of the work to accomplish the referencing task, and for this reason are called *referring expressions*. The elaborateness of referring expressions will depend on whether the audience knows what is being described, whether the referent being conjured up is present in the situation, and where in the discourse the expression occurs. Expressions that function to introduce an element are usually fuller than those that remention and thereby remind the reader about something that has already been introduced.

Researchers have studied the location and function of full expressions (full noun phrases), expressions that serve as reminders (anaphoric expressions, usually pronouns), and null expressions in which the referent is presupposed, but not referred to directly (zero anaphora). Also included in referencing analyses are expressions that do not refer to a specific element (indefinite referring expressions such as "a book") and general terms ("anyone"). Further, researchers have engaged in "participant tracking," wherein a particular referent in a segment of discourse is traced through the text to determine where, how, and how well it is described (with full noun phrases, with pronouns, or zero anaphor; Bennett-Kastor, 1983; Klecan-Aker, 1985), and what linguistic and cognitive factors govern its various forms (Hewitt, in press). Finally, researchers have studied referencing in clinical populations identifying instances of ambiguity and inappropriate use of referring expressions (Earle, 1983, Rochester & Martin, 1977; see Ulatowska et al., chapter 3, this volume, for a review of such studies in aphasia).

Local Level Cohesion Indicators. The rementioning of a particular element in a text not only helps the audience to know what is being talked about, but it has a second function—that of achieving discourse cohesion. Halliday and Hasan (1976), in their influential study of cohesion in discourse, described lexical reiteration, substitution, ellipsis, and various types of phoric referencing (referring to elements in the situation and to earlier or later elements in the text) as a way users of discourse weave nearby elements of the text together. The approach to cohesion taken by Halliday and Hasan and their followers (Coelho et al., chapter 6, this volume; Liles, 1985; Strong & Shaver, 1991) emphasizes local elements in a text, with a focus mostly on nominal referring expressions.

Local level but nonnominal cohesion markers studied by Halliday and Hasan and others (L. Bloom, Lahey, Hood, Lifter, & Fiess, 1980; Segal, Duchan, & Scott, 1991) are intersentential connectives. These connectives have been classified semantically as expressions of additive ("and," "or," "furthermore"), temporal ("then," "after," "next"), causal ("so," "because," "for this reason"), and adversative ("but," "however," "though," "nonetheless," "yet") (L. Bloom et al., 1980; Stein & Glenn, 1979. For an argument that these connectives may be serving a more global function rather than a local one, see Duchan et al., 1992; and Segal et al., 1991).

Global Level Indicators. Discourse structuring at the global level will be different for different types of discourse genres. Stories have been found to have a structure of multiple sentence units referred to as an *episode structure*;

conversations have a *topical structure*; lessons a *participant structure*; and conflict talk an *argument structure*. Global level analyses not only aim at discovering the larger constituents of discourse, but also the contour of those constituents in relation to one another. So a full global analysis for stories would not only depict the episode structure but how the episodes interconnect (e.g., related temporally, causally) and how they relate to the setting and ending.

Discourse analyses have examined text for indicators in the language of global structuring. For example, Young (1987) discovered a language of "edgework" in her adult storytellers that they use to indicate that they are moving from a conversational mode to a story, Schiffrin (1987) studied indicators of boundaries in adult arguments, and various researchers have found that intersentential connectives tie to global constituent boundaries in oral stories (Duchan et al., 1992; McCabe & Peterson, 1991; Segal et al., 1991).

Deictic Elements. Analysts of discourse often choose what to study for a particular segment of a discourse genre based on what is salient for all exemplars from that genre. So studies of stories tend to focus on the plot structure, studies of lessons on the didactic ways turns are exchanged, studies of event descriptions on the temporal and causal links of the subevents being depicted, and studies of verbal conflicts on the argument structure. What this single focus fails to capture is the multiple levels at which a discourse can be organized. Bruner (1986) argued that narratives, for example, have a dual landscape, one involving the logical plot structure, the landscape of action; and a second involving the felt experiences of those involved in the action, the landscape of consciousness.

Besides examining the surface meanings of discourse, one can, through discourse analysis, discover a more backgrounded meaning, that having to do with how the discourse is framed. For example, those engaged in discourse production and comprehension need to keep track of where and when the events are taking place, and from whose perspective it is told. My colleagues and I have been studying such framing for narrative discourse under the rubric of "deictic centering" (Duchan, Bruder, & Hewitt, in press). We have put forward the thesis that typical narrative (not the writing of modernist authors such as Virginia Woolf) cast their story in a coherent time and space, and usually from a particular person's point of view. So deictic terms in a story can originate with the character from whose perspective the story is being told (e.g., "I," "you"). Similarly, stories are told with spatial and temporal centering so that spatial deictic terms ("come," "go," "here," "there") and temporal terms ("now," "then," "yesterday") take their meaning from the established deictic center. Also implicated in the deictic structuring of discourse are linguistic devices that designate movement from one place to another, disjunctures in time, and shifts from the objective to the subjective worlds of one character or from one character's subjective experience to that of another. Deictic shifts such as these can be signaled by many linguistic devices such as adverbs, preposed adverbials, connectives indicating disjuncture, perception verbs indicating subjective experience, and others (Zubin & Hewitt, in press).

Genre Framing. Discourse analyses have been designed to discover unique characteristics of different discourse genres. The most commonly studied genres are narratives, lessons, and conversations. Other genres such as joint problem solving (Domingo, chapter 7, this volume), expository (Westby, 1989), persuasive talk (Weiss & Sacks, 1991), interviews (Mishler, 1984), courtroom discourse (Barry, 1991), and conflict talk (Grimshaw, 1990) comprise a healthy and important subset of contributions to our understanding of discourse.

Summary. This section has presented various linguistic approaches to the study of discourse structure. The review has shown how the language of the text is implicated in conveying discourse information at five different discourse levels. (See Table 1.1 for summary outline.)

FUTURE DIRECTIONS

The contributors to this volume have taken an important step in offering ways for studying discourse of typical as well as atypical adults. They provide a translation of some of the various methods available for analyzing discourse to the study of the everyday communication of adults with different sorts of communication disorders. The approach is normative where discourse of typical adults of different ages is taken to be a standard against which those with communication disorders

TABLE 1.1
Levels of Discourse, Linguistic Indicators of Discourse Structure, and Functions Carried Out at Each Level

	Discourse Structuring	
Level	*Linguistic Indicators*	*Functions*
Referring expressions	Nouns, noun phrases definite & indef determiners, full NP vs Pronouns	Introduce and maintain elements, track participants
Local relations	Word order, grammatical forms, referring expressions	Create local cohesion
Global relations	Connectives, paragraph markers, silence	Identify global structure
Deictic structure	Lexical indicators perception verbs, assuming anothers' voice	Indicate point of view Mark frame shifts
Genre	Framing phrases macrostructuring	Inform, persuade, describe, entertain, participate, teach

are compared. The results bring us closer to understanding what can go wrong in discourse use, and thus provides us with a beginning for developing discourse-based language intervention techniques.

Also needed for a fully developed understanding of discourse in those with language disorders is a view of how that discourse is structured on its own terms. That is, discourse can also be treated as an idiolect, where the patterns in the abnormal discourse are studied for their regularities. Borrowing from the work on cross-cultural linguistics, one might develop ways of looking at an individual's discourse within a particular genre. For example, Michaels (1981) and Heath (1983) found that children created what was considered by those from a different culture to be inappropriately organized stories. Detailed examination revealed unexpected competencies underlying those unaccepted stories, and allowed for a more positive approach to helping them develop discourse compatible with the classroom culture. The work of Gee (1991), Duchan (1994), and Hewitt, Duchan, and Segal (in press) suggest the profitability of looking at unconventional discourse for what it contains rather than to focus solely on what is missing.

A final and crucial area of investigation of those using unconventional discourse is to develop ways in which that discourse can become more acceptable with training. An added contribution to the efforts of the authors in this volume would be to learn, with further research, that the discourse differences of these clinic populations can become less different with discourse therapies. But that effort requires another set of studies and another book. This book has brought us much closer to that possibility.

REFERENCES

Almeida, M. (in press). Time in narratives. In J. Duchan, G. Bruder, & L. Hewitt (Eds.), *Deixis in narrative: A cognitive science perspective.* Hillsdale, NJ: Lawrence Erlbaum Associates.

Bakhtin, M. (1985). *The dialogic imagination.* Austin, TX: University of Texas Press.

Bamberg, M. (1991). Conceptualization via narrative: A discussion of Donald E. Polkinghorne's "Narrative and self concept." *Journal of Narrative and Life History, 1,* 155–167.

Bamberg, M., & Damrad-Frye, R. (1991). On the ability to provide evaluative comments: Further explorations of children's narrative competencies. *Journal of Child Language, 18,* 689–710.

Barry, A. (1991). Narrative style and witness testimony. *Journal of Narrative and Life History, 1,* 281–293.

Bartlett, F. (1932). *Remembering: An experimental and social study.* New York: Cambridge University Press.

Bedrosian, J., & Prutting, C. (1978). Communicative performance of mentally retarded adults in four conversational settings. *Journal of Speech and Hearing Research, 21,* 79–95.

Bennett-Kastor, T. (1983). Noun phrases and coherence in child narratives. *Journal of Child Language, 10,* 135–149.

Bloom, L., Lahey, M., Hood, K., Lifter, K., & Fiess, K. (1980). Complex sentences: Acquisition of syntactic connectives and the semantic relations they encode. *Journal of Child Language, 7,* 235–262.

Bloom, R., Borod, J., Obler, L., & Gerstman, L. (1992). Impact of emotional content on discourse production in patients with unilateral brain damage. *Brain and Language, 42*, 153–164.

Brewer, W., & Lichtenstein, E. (1982). Stories are to entertain: A structural-affect theory of stories. *Journal of Pragmatics, 6*, 473–486.

Bruner, J. (1986). *Actual minds, possible worlds*. Cambridge, MA: Harvard University Press.

Cazden, C. (1988). *Classroom discourse*. Portsmouth, NH: Heinemann.

Chafe, W. (Ed.). (1980). *The pear stories: Cognitive, cultural and linguistic aspects of narrative production*. Norwood, NJ: Ablex.

Chafe, W. (1985). Linguistic differences produced by differences between speaking and writing. In D. Olson, N. Torrance, & A. Hildyard (Eds.), *Literacy, language and learning: The nature and consequences of reading and writing* (pp. 105–123). New York: Cambridge University Press.

Clifford, J. (1983). On ethnographic authority. *Representations, 1*, 118–146.

Clifford, J. (1988). *The predicament of culture: Twentieth century ethnography, literature, and art*. Cambridge, MA: Harvard University Press.

Crago, M., & Eriks-Brophy, A. (1994). Culture, conversation, and interaction: Implications for intervention. In J. Duchan, L. Hewitt, & R. Sonnenmeier (Eds.), *Pragmatics: From theory to practice*. Englewood Cliffs, NJ: Prentice-Hall.

Drew, P. (1984). Speakers' reportings in invitation sequences. In J. Atkinson & J. Heritage (Eds.), *Structures of social action: Studies in conversation analysis* (pp. 129–151). New York: Cambridge University Press.

Drew, P., & Heritage, J. (1992). *Talk at work*. New York: Cambridge University Press.

Duchan, J. (1994). Intervention principles for gestalt-style learners. In J. Duchan, L. Hewitt, & R. Sonnenmeier (Eds.), *Pragmatics from theory to practice* (pp. 149–163). Englewood Cliffs, NJ: Prentice-Hall.

Duchan, J., Bruder, G., & Hewitt, J. (Eds.). (In press). *Deixis in narrative: A cognitive science perspective*. Hillsdale, NJ: Lawrence Erlbaum Associates.

Duchan, J., Meth, M., & Waltzman, D. (1992). "Then" as an indicator of deictic discontinuity in adults' oral descriptions of a film. *Journal of Speech and Hearing Research, 35*, 1367–1375.

Earle, C. (1983). *Confusion resulting from misreferencing: A case study of a language/learning disabled adult*. Unpublished master's thesis, State University of New York at Buffalo, NY.

Frederiksen, C., Bracewell, R., Breuleux, A., & Renauld, A. (1990). The cognitive representation and processing of discourse: Function and dysfunction. In Y. Joanette & H. Brownell (Eds.), *Discourse ability and brain damage: Theoretical and empirical perspectives* (pp. 69–110). New York: Springer-Verlag.

Gee, J. (1991). A linguistic approach to narrative. *Journal of Narrative and Life History, 1*, 15–39.

Gee, J. (1992). *The social mind*. New York: Bergin & Garvey.

Geertz, C. (Ed.). (1988). *Works and lives: The anthropologist as author*. Stanford, CA: Stanford University Press.

Goodwin, C. (1981). *Conversational organization: Interaction between speakers and hearers*. New York: Academic Press.

Grimes, J. (1975). *The thread of discourse*. The Hague: Mouton.

Grimshaw, A. (Ed.). (1990). *Conflict talk*. New York: Cambridge University Press.

Halliday, M., & Hasan, R. (1976). *Cohesion in English*. New York: Longman.

Haviland, J., & Goldston, R. (in press). Emotion and narrative: The agony and ecstasy. In K. Strongman (Ed.), *International review of studies in emotion* (Vol. 2). New York: Wiley.

Heath, S. B. (1983). *Ways with words*. New York: Cambridge University Press.

Hewitt, L. (in press). Reduced anaphor in subjective contexts in narrative fiction. In J. Duchan, G. Bruder, & L. Hewitt (Eds.), *Deixis in narrative: A cognitive science perspective*. Hillsdale, NJ: Lawrence Erlbaum Associates.

Hewitt, L., Duchan, J., & Segal, E. (in press). Structure and function of verbal conflicts among adults with mental retardation. *Discourse Processes*.

Higginbotham, J. (1989). The interplay of communication device output mode and interaction style between nonspeaking persons and their speaking partners. *Journal of Speech and Hearing Disorders, 54*, 320–333.

Hobbs, J. (1990). *Literature and cognition.* Stanford, CA: Center for the Study of Language and Information.

Hopper, P. (1979). Aspect and foregrounding in discourse. In T. Givon (Ed.), *Syntax and semantics* (Vol. 12, pp. 213–241). New York: Academic Press.

Hudson, J., Gebelt, J., Haviland, J., & Bentivenga, C. (1992). Emotion and narrative structure in young children's personal accounts. *Journal of Narrative and Life History, 2*, 129–150.

Joanette, Y., & Brownell, H. (1990). *Discourse ability and brain damage: Theoretical and empirical perspectives.* New York: Springer-Verlag.

Kemper, S., & Edwards, L. (1986). Children's expression of causality and their construction of narratives. *Topics in Language Disorders, 7*, 11–20.

Klecan-Aker, J. (1985). Syntactic abilities in normal and language-deficient middle school children. *Topics in Language Disorders, 5*, 46–54.

Labov, W. (1984). Intensity. In D. Schiffrin (Ed.), *Meaning, form, and use in context: Linguistic applications* (pp. 43–70). Washington, DC: Georgetown University Press.

Labov, W., & Fanshel, D. (1977). *Therapeutic discourse: Psychotherapy as conversation.* New York: Academic Press.

Labov, W., & Waletsky, J. (1967). Narrative analysis: Oral versions of personal experience. In J. Helms (Ed.), *Essays on the verbal and visual arts* (pp. 12–44). Seattle: University of Washington Press.

Liles, B. (1985). Cohesion in the narratives of normal and language-disordered children. *Journal of Speech and Hearing Research, 28*, 123–133.

Mandler, J. (1984). *Stories, scripts, and scenes: Aspects of schema theory.* Hillsdale, NJ: Lawrence Erlbaum Associates.

Mandler, J., & Johnson, N. (1977). Remembrance of things parsed: Story structure and recall. *Cognitive Psychology, 9*, 111–151.

Marshall, J. (1977). Disorders in the expression of language. In M. Morton & J. Marshall (Eds.), *Psycholinguistics: Developmental and pathological.* Ithaca, NY: Cornell University Press.

Maynard, D. (1992). On clinicians co-implicating recipients' perspective in the delivery of diagnostic news. In P. Drew & J. Heritage (Ed.), *Talk at work* (pp. 331–358). New York: Cambridge University Press.

McCabe, A., & Peterson, C. (Eds.). (1991). *Developing narrative structure* (pp. 43–58). Hillsdale, NJ: Lawrence Erlbaum Associates.

Mehan, H. (1979). *Learning lessons: Social organization in the classroom.* Cambridge, MA: Harvard University Press.

Michaels, S. (1981). Sharing time: Children's narrative styles and differential access to literacy. *Language in Society, 10*, 423–442.

Mishler, E. (1984). *The discourse of medicine: Dialectics of medical interviews.* Norwood, NJ: Ablex.

Nelson, K. (Ed.). (1986). *Event knowledge.* Hillsdale, NJ: Lawrence Erlbaum Associates.

Reilly, J. (1992). How to tell a good story: The intersection of language and affect in children's narratives. *Journal of Narrative and Life History, 1*, 355–377.

Rochester, S., & Martin, J. (1977). The art of referring: The speaker's use of noun phrases to instruct the listener. In R. Freedle (Ed.), *Discourse production and comprehension.* Norwood, NJ: Ablex.

Rosenau, P. (1992). *Post-modernism and the social sciences.* Princeton, NJ: Princeton University Press.

Rumelhart, D. (1975). Notes on a schema for stories. In D. Brobrow & A. Collins (Eds.), *Representation and understanding: Studies in cognitive science* (pp. 211–236). New York: Academic Press.

Schank, R., & Abelson, R. (1977). *Scripts, plans, goals, and understanding.* Hillsdale, NJ: Lawrence Erlbaum Associates.

Schegloff, E., Jefferson, G., & Sacks, H. (1977). The preference for self-correction in the organization of repair for conversation. *Language, 53*, 361–82.

Schiffrin, D. (1987). *Discourse markers*. New York: Cambridge University Press.

Segal, E., Duchan, J., & Scott, P. (1991). The role of interclausal connectives in narrative structuring: Evidence from adults' interpretations of simple stories. *Discourse Processes, 14*, 27–54.

Shatz, M., & Gelman, R. (1973). The development of communication skills. In *Monographs of the Society for Research in Child Development, 38* (5, Serial No. 152).

Stein, N., & Glenn, C. (1979). An analysis of story comprehension in elementary school children. In R. Freedle (Ed.), *New directions in discourse processing* (pp. 53–120). Norwood, NJ: Ablex.

Strong, C., & Shaver, J. (1991). Stability of cohesion in the spoken narratives of language-impaired and normally developing school-aged children. *Journal of Speech and Hearing Research, 34*, 95–111.

Tannen, D. (1985). Relative focus on involvement in oral and written discourse. In D. Olson, N. Torrance, & A. Hildyard (Eds.), *Literacy, language and learning: The nature and consequences of reading and writing* (pp. 124–147). New York: Cambridge University Press.

Trabasso, T., Secco, T., & van den Broek, P. (1984). Causal cohesion and story coherence. In H. Mandl, N. Stein, & T. Trabasso (Eds.), *Learning and comprehension of text* (pp. 147–165). Hillsdale, NJ: Lawrence Erlbaum Associates.

van Dijk, T., & Kintsch, W. (1983). *Strategies of discourse comprehension*. New York: Academic Press.

Weiss, D., & Sacks, J. (1991). Persuasive strategies used by preschool children. *Discourse Processes, 14*, 55–72.

Westby, C. (1985). Learning to talk—talking to learn: Oral-literate language differences. In C. Simon (Ed.), *Communication skills and classroom success: Therapy methodologies for language-learning disabled students* (pp. 181–218). San Diego, CA: College Hill Press.

Westby, C. (1989). Assessing and remediating text comprehension problems. In A. Kamhi & H. Catts (Eds.), *Reading disabilities: A developmental language perspective* (pp. 199–259). Boston: Little, Brown.

White, H. (1981). The value of narrativity in the representation of reality. In J. Mitchell (Ed.), *On narrative* (pp. 35–75). Chicago, IL: University of Chicago Press.

Young, K. (1987). *Taleworlds and storyrealms: The phenomenology of narrative*. Boston, MA: Martinus Nijhoff.

Young, K. (1991). Perspectives on embodiment: The uses of narrativity in ethnographic writing. *Journal of Narrative and Life History, 1*, 213–243.

Zubin, D., & Hewitt, L. (in press). Linguistic devices for spatial and temporal tracking. In J. Duchan, G. Bruder, & L. Hewitt (Eds.), *Deixis in narrative: A cognitive science perspective*. Hillsdale, NJ: Lawrence Erlbaum Associates.

Chapter 2

Intersubject Variability in Adult Normal Discourse

Loraine K. Obler
The City University of New York Graduate School
Boston University School of Medicine
and
Boston VA Medical Center

Rhoda Au
Boston University School of Medicine
and
Boston VA Medical Center

Jay Kugler
University of Chicago

Janis Melvold
Michael Tocco
Martin L. Albert
Boston University School of Medicine
and
Boston VA Medical Center

In order to evaluate discourse parameters of patients with brain damage, one requires data on normal discourse behavior. Yet there is very little literature on the discourse characteristics of normal adult individuals, and what there is, at least in the elderly population, provides several points of controversy (Bayles & Kaszniak, 1987). For example, some studies show more elaborate discourse with aging (Obler & Albert, 1984), whereas others report less complex speech (Kemper, 1987a; Kynette & Kemper, 1986). Some report higher quality narratives with age (Kemper, Rash, Kynette, & Norman, 1990), whereas others report lower quality (Ehrlich, 1990; North, Ulatowska, Macaluso-Haynes, & Bell, 1986; Ulatowska, Cannito, Hayashi, & Fleming, 1986). In this chapter we argue that these controversies arise as the result of methodological issues, and in particular from an inherent variability among individual discourse "styles" that may increase with age.

We review first the studies that report a decline in discourse abilities with age. For example, on a task of producing procedural discourse, subjects were asked to describe the processes involved in mailing a letter, polishing shoes, and shopping. Elderly subjects produced fewer propositions conveying essential steps, and their anaphoric pronoun usage became more ambiguous, despite the fact that this was a group with more years of education than average (North et al., 1986). In Ulatowska et al. (1986) the same research team elaborated on this finding of referential ambiguity, noting that some decline was seen in the young elderly (with a mean age of approximately 70 years), but more was seen in the older elderly (with a mean age of approximately 82.3 years). Ehrlich (1990) confirmed these findings in a picture description narrative task with individuals with somewhat fewer (M = 11.8) years of education, as did Glosser and Deser (1992) who compared middle aged (M = 52) to elderly (M = 76) adults.

In their 1989 study, Kemper and colleagues reported fewer complex (left-branching) syntactic structures in older adults. They also noted decreased fluency in elderly individuals; for example, the proportion of discourse consisting of sentence fragments and lexical fillers was greater. In this same study, however, readers rated the discourse of the older subjects as being clearer and more interesting than that of the younger controls. Elsewhere, Kemper et al. (1990) reported that older subjects are most likely to achieve what they consider to be the highest levels of discourse production, in that they include morals in their stories.

In the Glosser and Deser (1992) paper the authors studied lexical errors, syntactic complexity, lexical cohesion, and thematic coherence in interviews among their middle-aged (M = 52) and elderly (M = 76) healthy subjects. Although they observed a decline in the thematic coherence of elders, they found no age differences for the linguistic measures at the lexical and syntactic levels.

It is worth noting that Glosser and Deser reported no differences in neurolinguistic aspects of discourse (these include lexical and syntactic performance), or even on the macrolinguistic measure of lexical coherence across contiguous sentences. Such reporting of lack of differences is rare in the literature on discourse in aging. What also does not get emphasized or, often, reported in the published literature, however, are instances in which significant differences may arise between, say, a group of subjects in their 30s and another in their 60s, but not between the 30s group and one of subjects in their 70s. One would, of course, have expected 70-year-olds to be even more advanced in whatever performance distinguished the 30-year-olds and the 60-year-olds.

The failure to report "no-difference" data can be attributed to some biases in how science is conducted, whereby findings of "no difference" between groups are considered to be inherently less interesting, and thus less publishable, than findings of difference. Of course the no-difference findings may in fact reflect lack of differences, but the scientists reporting them may also be suspected of not having asked the right questions that would reveal differences (Type 2 errors).

The fact that scientists reporting differences may have asked questions in such a way as to appear to obtain what are in fact spurious differences (Type 1 errors) is deemed less problematic in modern science. Findings of nonlinear differences go unreported for more subtle reasons, in our experience. This is because it is hard to explain them, and researchers may be reluctant to publish findings that they cannot explain.

Over the years the Language in the Aging Brain Laboratory at the Boston VA Medical Center has conducted a series of analyses of the microtexture of oral discourse, as part of a longitudinal study of language changes associated with aging. What we have been most impressed with is the lack of consistent age-related findings for discourse phenomena. In this chapter we focus specifically and by choice on these aspects of aging research often omitted in the literature: findings of no differences for groups, and nonlinear significant variations. We then attempt to explain these findings that are often referred to as "absence of findings."

We present next a set of data summarized by Kugler (1990) derived from the initial Language in the Aging Brain Laboratory testing of 160 subjects ages 30–79. Men and women were included as normal subjects in equal proportion if they had no history of psychiatric illness, alcoholism, neurological illness, learning disability, uncorrected hearing loss, or vision loss. Additional information on these subjects is available in Obler, Au, and Albert (in press); for our purposes it is worth noting that the average education of the population is about 14 years.

In the course of a 4-hour battery of tests, subjects were asked to describe the Cookie Theft picture from the Boston Diagnostic Aphasia Examination (Goodglass & Kaplan, 1972). Subjects' responses were taped and transcribed. In addition to the eight semantic/thematic items, fillers were counted, word counts were made, parts of speech were coded, indefinite references were tabulated, comments were noted (including judgments, unsureness, personalization, and apologies), and repetitions were counted, both verbatim and nonverbatim. Parts of speech were counted in their specifics and in terms of the superordinate categories of functor versus substantive. In addition, the (relatively rare) errors were counted: omissions, paragrammatisms, and semantic and verbal paraphasias.

Subjects had been selected from four age groups: 30–39, 50–59, 60–69, and 70–79. Comparing the potential differences across the four age groups, using both parametric and nonparametric statistics as appropriate, we found no age differences for the following variables: number of themes, number of words per theme, repetitions, usage of all parts of speech (with the exception of adverbs), and use of fillers. (Note that for these analyses, outliers' data were excluded. They came from three subjects in their 70s, one in the 60s, but no one in the 30s or 50s.)

Where differences were found, on the remaining variables, the pattern was never linear. Consider, for example, the use of the eight themes. There was a significant age-related difference in one: The mother was oblivious or not paying attention to what was going on (see Fig. 2.1). Significant group differences (*p*

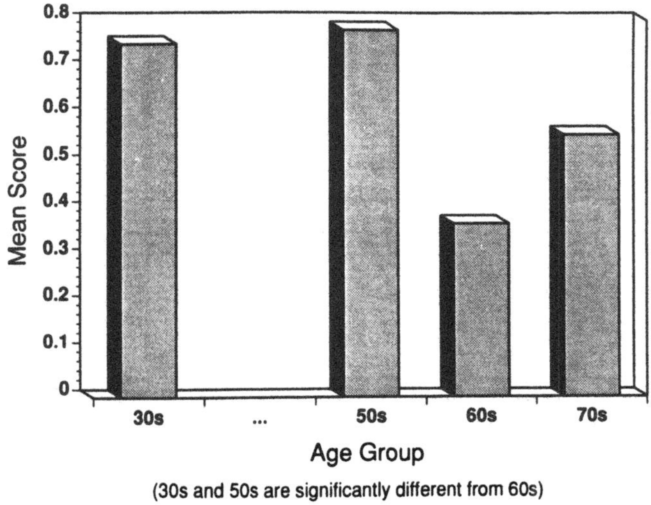

FIG. 2.1. Oral cookie theft picture (subjects mention that the mother is oblivious).

< .003) were found whereby the subjects in their 30s and those in their 50s were more likely to mention this theme than were those in their 60s ($p < .05$). Subjects in their 70s commented on this fact an intermediate number of times. (Note that no differences were seen on the remaining seven themes.)

On word omissions there was a significant group effect ($p < .05$) whereby the 60-year-olds performed worse then the 30-year-olds ($p < .05$) (see Fig. 2.2). The performance of the 50s and 70s was intermediate, and did not differ significantly from that of any other group.

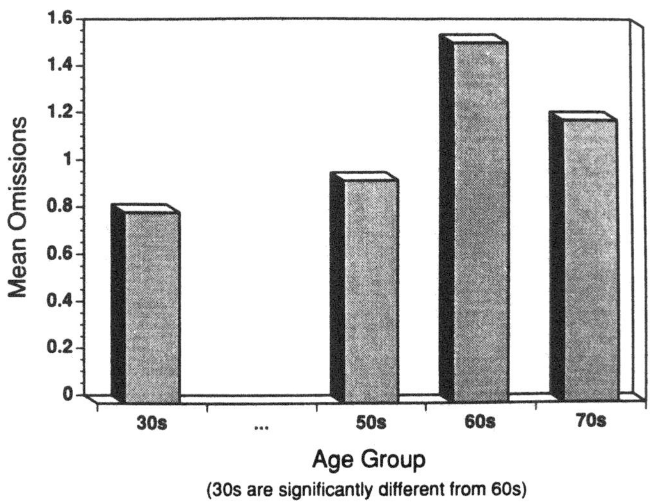

FIG. 2.2. Oral cookie theft picture (omissions).

A third measure of groups' errors for semantic paraphasias approached significance ($p = .06$; see Fig. 2.3). Because it was so close to significant, we performed post hoc group comparisons in order not to overreport absence of differences. In this instance, it was not the 60-year-olds but the 30-year-olds who made the most errors. The 30s produced more semantic paraphasias than the 50s who gave fewest ($p < .05$). This somewhat different U-curve is difficult to explain; in this instance it was our examiner's post hoc impression that the subjects in their 30s were rushing, and, for example, would often say "chair" for "stool." For the subjects in their 60s and 70s, by contrast, paraphasias appear to have resulted from problems with lexical access, as indicated by pausing, self-corrections, and frank statements about their difficulty in finding the words they were looking for.

The age groups differed significantly on the measure of the ratio of substantives per total words ($p = .004$). The pattern of significance was different from those just reported, in this instance the subjects in their 30s and those in their 70s produced significantly fewer substantives per word than did those in their 50s and 60s ($p < .05$; see Fig. 2.4). Note that Tocco (1990), by contrast, reported no significant finding for what one would expect to be a related measure: words per theme (see Fig. 2.5).

In a second set of analyses, we analyzed the data with no exclusion of outliers in order to fully represent the heterogeneity of the elderly. To determine the range of performance, we selected, for each age cell, the lowest and highest scores for individual variables. Because we focus on the range of behavior in the following analyses, these statistics are descriptive.

Consider the range of total words in response to the Cookie Theft picture (see Fig. 2.6). Note that the range is great for the 30-year-olds and the 50-year-olds and even greater for the 60-year-olds and the 70-year-olds. A similar pattern is

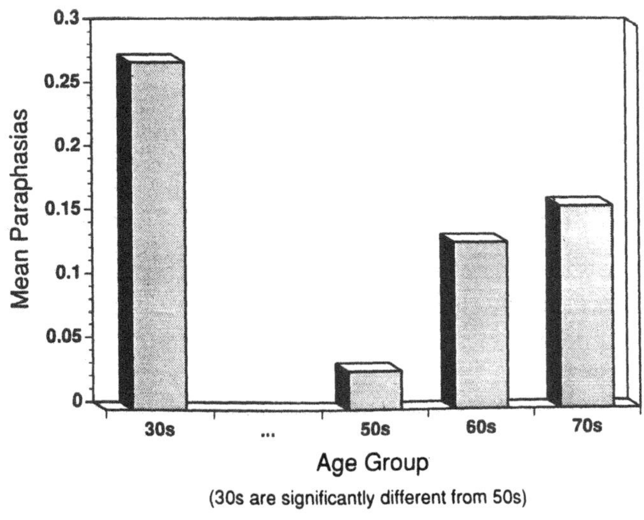

FIG. 2.3. Oral cookie theft picture (semantic paraphasias).

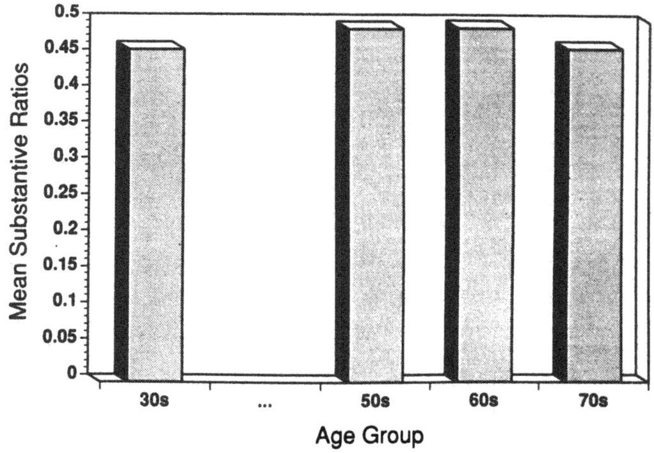

(30s and 70s are significantly different from 50s and 60s)

FIG. 2.4. Oral cookie theft picture (substantives per words).

seen for the measure of words per theme (see Fig. 2.7). This arises because the number of themes reported does not change significantly with age on this task. All groups ranged from including five to eight out of the eight possible themes.

In Fig. 2.8, note that although there was a tendency for the older subjects to have fewer perfect scores (i.e., scores of 8 points) there was a broad range for all age groups.

As to the fillers (Fig. 2.9), all age groups contained individuals who did not produce any. Moreover, there was some increase with age group in the high

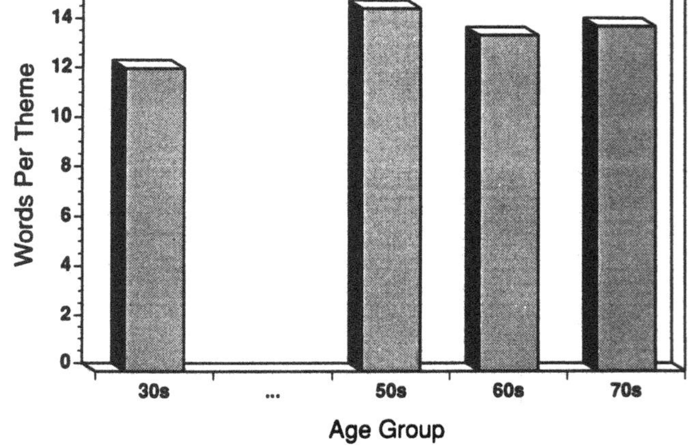

FIG. 2.5. Oral cookie theft picture (words per theme).

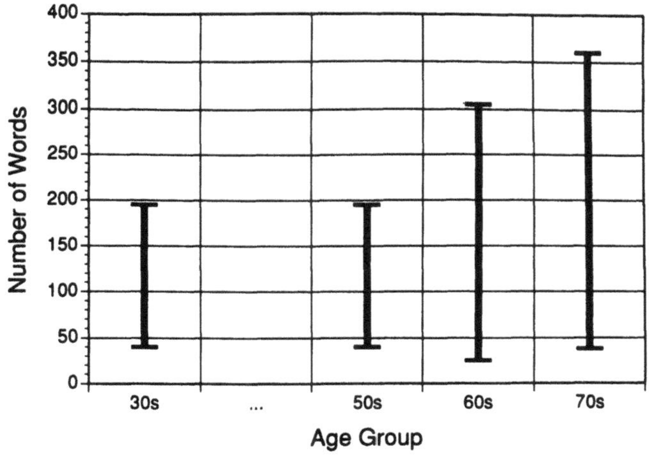

FIG. 2.6. Oral cookie theft picture (range of total words).

number of fillers produced (the 30-year-olds produced 8; the 50- and 60-year-olds produced 13, and the 70-year olds produced 20).

Next, let us look at the measures for indefinite words (Fig. 2.10) and mentions of unsureness (e.g., "Oh, what is that called?"; Fig. 2.11). For both these measures there was a relatively small range, with individuals in each age group who produced none. The 60-year-olds achieved the highest score for unsureness and the 50-year-olds had the highest score for indefinite words.

Results from the sum of extra-story content elements were similar (this score consisted of the number of judgments plus personalization, statements of unsureness, and apologies). Again, the range was similar for all age groups (see Fig. 2.12).

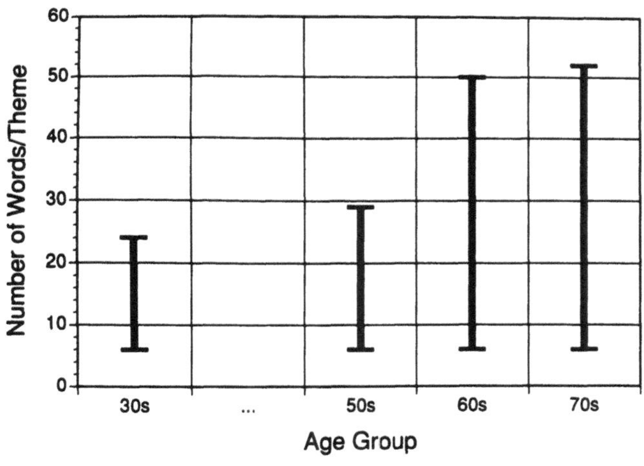

FIG. 2.7. Oral cookie theft picture (words per theme).

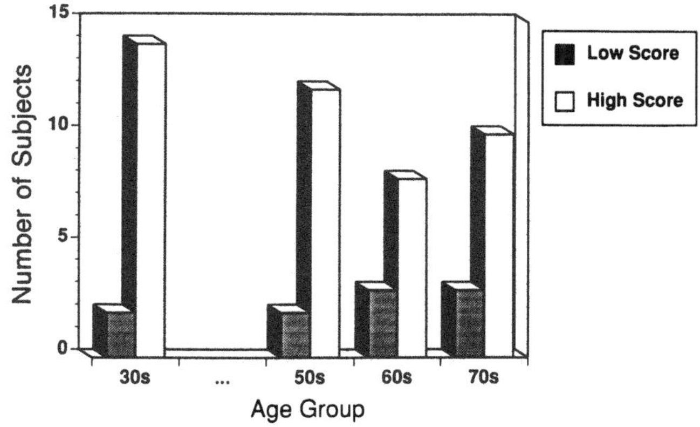

FIG. 2.8. Oral cookie theft story items. Numbers of subjects scoring lowest [5] and highest [8].

DISCUSSION

Clearly, there is a great deal of variability in discourse texture in every adult age decade we have studied. On only one measure—narrative length—can we point to marked increase in variability with age. On most other measures, equal degrees of variability are seen within each decade. One might argue that our substantial findings of "no age-related difference" in these microlinguistic discourse phenomena results from our choice of phenomena to be measured. We would respond that, for these phenomena, our various modes of analysis suggest that there indeed seem to be no age-related differences that approach the interindividual ones. One might also argue that our measures were too coarse—or too refined—to reveal

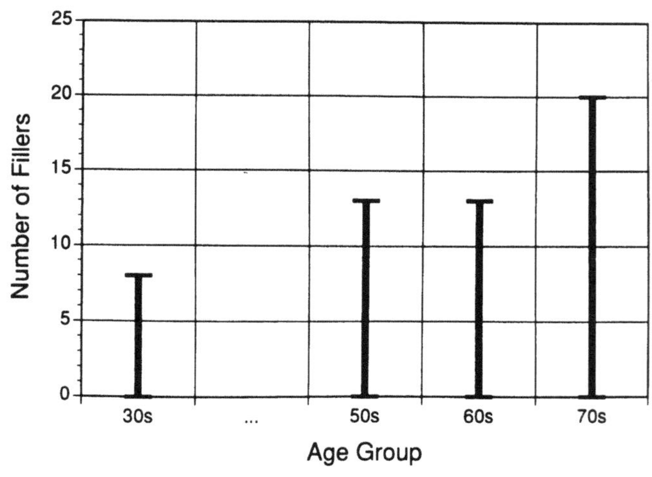

FIG. 2.9. Oral cookie theft picture (filler usage for men and women).

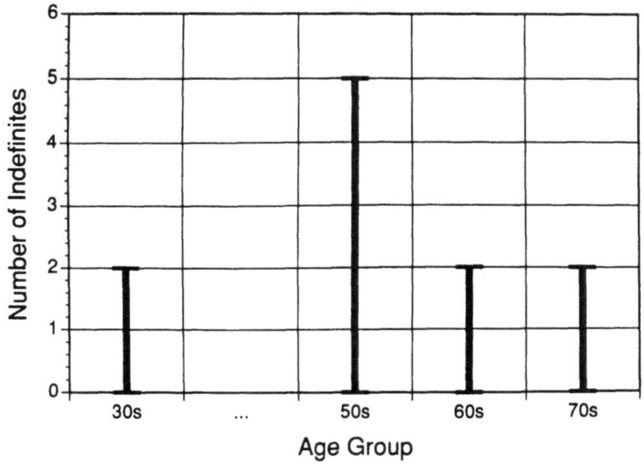

FIG. 2.10. Oral cookie theft picture (use of indefinites).

true age-related differences. Our response would be that although replication of the studies using different measures could perhaps be useful, other similar studies, such as the study of Glosser and Deser (1992), corroborated our results by also finding no age-related differences on similar measures.

Serious methodological issues are raised by these findings. These complement those mentioned in De Santi and Obler (1991). In previous publications (Obler & Albert, 1980), we have suggested that the narrative task employed has important consequences for whether or not age-related differences are seen on discourse studies involving memory (most markedly paragraph recall tasks). The decline in the number of themes or propositions is seen on such tasks as the Wechsler

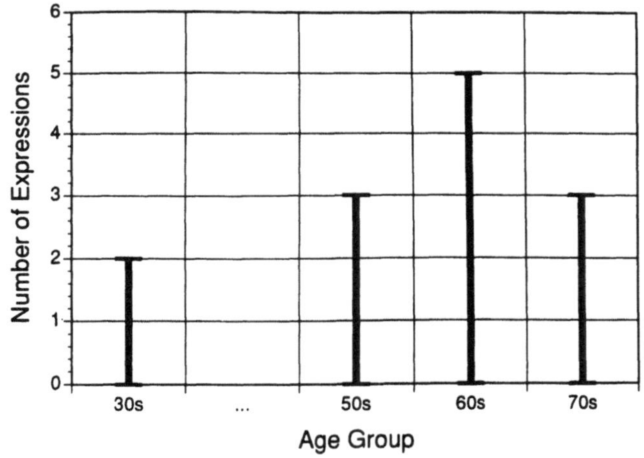

FIG. 2.11. Oral cookie theft picture (expressions of unsureness).

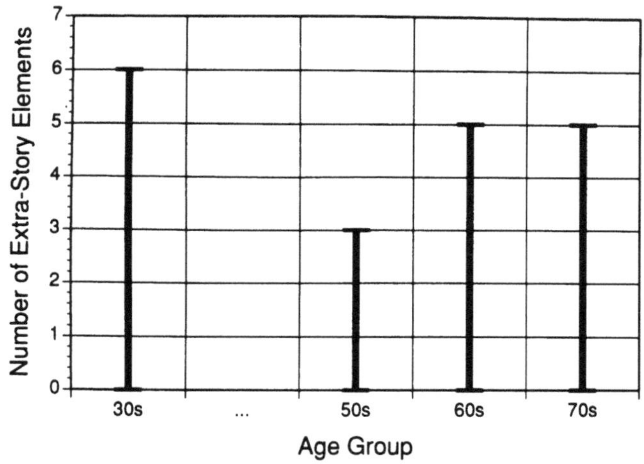

FIG. 2.12. Oral cookie theft picture (sum of extra-story elements).

Logical Memory Task, a story-recall task (Obler & Albert, 1980); even telling the story of Little Red Riding Hood evidences this decline (Tocco, 1990), although this is a task requiring long-term rather than short-term memory. By contrast, on the task of looking at the Cookie Theft picture and describing it, where memory did not come into play, no such decline is seen.

In this chapter we point out two other methodological factors that have consequences for what is reported in studies of language in normal aging. One is the extent to which items counted are reported in absolute numbers, rather than as a proportion of the total. Our most striking example of a finding that would be reported differently comes from our study of the Little Red Riding Hood data (Tocco, 1990). Here, in a subsequent test session, we taped and transcribed the same healthy normal subjects who had participated in the first test sessions, now telling the Little Red Riding Hood story. After reviewing half of the subjects' stories, we made a list of 26 thematic elements that occur in that story in chronological order, beginning with "Little Red Riding Hood was a girl with a red cloak" and ending with "They all lived happily ever after." To consider the temporal sequencing of thematic elements, we matched each subject's theme order to the list of 26 story elements, assigning the appropriate number from the baseline list to each proposition in the subject's response. Sequencing errors were then counted; they were defined as clauses having a temporal order number lower than the preceding number. Although the age-related pattern was not significant, the result of this analysis exhibited a linear decrease of sequencing errors with age (see Fig. 2.13). However, when we corrected for the number of themes produced, because the older subjects produced fewer themes overall (see Fig. 2.14), the ratio of sequencing errors per theme resulted in no age-related differences (see Fig. 2.15).

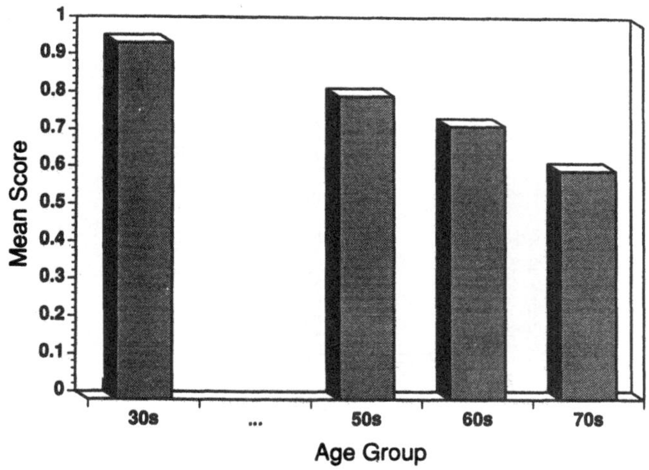

FIG. 2.13. Little Red Riding Hood (sequencing errors).

A second point of methodological importance is the potential difference that exclusion of outliers makes. As this practice is a standard technique in reporting the results of psychological experimentation, it is important to observe how many outliers are excluded from each age group. Our experience reported here leads us to expect that more outliers may be excluded among the older population. If so, this increasing variability is itself of interest for appreciating the range of normal behavior associated with aging.

A third methodological point recommends the use of more than two age groups—one younger and one older—in any study of aging. Although one increases the chances of finding nonlinear differences across groups if one employs three or more age groups, such findings presumably reflect the truths

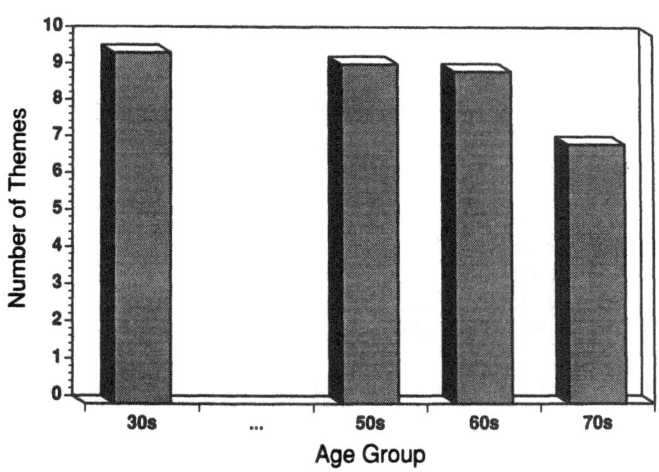

FIG. 2.14. Little Red Riding Hood (themes).

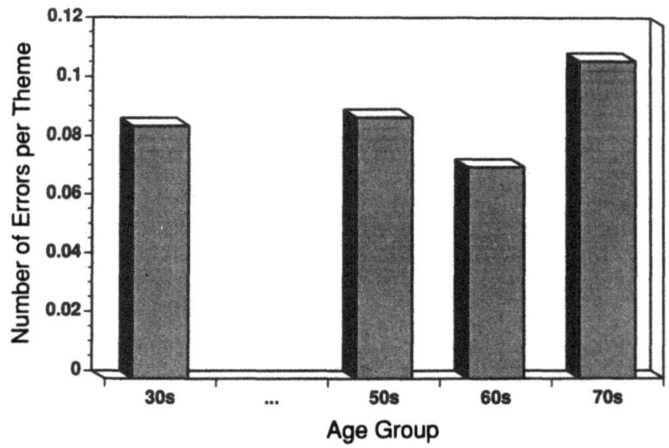

FIG. 2.15. Little Red Riding Hood (sequencing errors per theme).

about aging, and result in fewer Type 1 errors (i.e., reporting phenomena as different that are not really different).

Finally, we must discuss the clinical use of our conclusions about variability in normal discourse for studies of brain-damaged populations. Although some studies of discourse in brain-damaged populations employ a control group in order to learn what discourse in normal age- and education-matched adults looks like, many others do not, simply assuming that the types of errors seen in brain-damaged patients are not seen in normal adults. Studies such as those conducted in the Cross-Language Agrammatism series (Menn & Obler, 1990a), however, consistently demonstrate that there is overlap between the speech errors of normal adults and errors construed as aphasic in an aphasic population (Menn & Obler, 1990b). For that reason we recommend comparing the performance of a control group whenever the discourse of any clinical population is studied. Moreover, considering the variability reported in this chapter, we strongly suggest selection of large control groups for each cohort studied, so that the range of normal behavior within a given age interval can be determined.

REFERENCES

Bayles, K., & Kaszniak, A. (1987). *Communication and cognition in normal aging and dementia.* Boston, MA: College-Hill Press.

De Santi, S., & Obler, L. K. (1991). Methodological issues in the study of communication in the elderly. In D. Ripich (Ed.), *Handbook of geriatric communication disorders* (pp. 133–141). Austin, TX: Pro-Ed Series.

Ehrlich, J. (1990). *Influence of structure on the content of oral narrative in adults with dementia of the Alzheimer's type.* Unpublished doctoral dissertation, CUNY.

Glosser, G., & Deser, T. (1992). A comparison of changes on macrolinguisitic and microlinguistic aspects of discourse production on normal aging. *Journal of Gerontology: Psychological Sciences, 47,* 266–272.

Goodglass, H., & Kaplan, E. (1972). *The assessment of aphasia and related disorders*. Philadelphia: Febiger.

Kemper, S. (1987a). Life-span changes in syntactic complexity. *Journal of Gerontology, 42*, 232–238.

Kemper, S. (1987b). Syntactic complexity and the recall of prose by middle-aged and elderly adults. *Experimental Aging Research, 13*, 47–52.

Kemper, S., Rash, S., Kynette, D., & Norman, S. (1990). Telling stories: The structure of adults' narratives. *European Journal of Cognitive Psychology, 2*, 205–278.

Kynette, D., & Kemper, S. (1986). Aging and the loss of grammatical forms: A cross-sectional study of language performance. *Language and Communication, 6*, 43–49.

Kugler, J., 1990. [Unpublished data write-up].

Menn, L., & Obler, L. K. (Eds.). (1990a). *Agrammatic aphasia: A cross-language narrative sourcebook* (3 vols.). Amsterdam: Benjamins.

Menn, L., & Obler, L. K. (1990b). Cross-language data and theories of agrammatism. In L. Menn & L. K. Obler (Eds.), *Agrammatic aphasia: A cross-language narrative sourcebook* (Vol. 2, pp. 1369–1389). Amsterdam: Benjamins.

North, A., Ulatowska, H., Macaluso-Haynes, S., & Bell, H. (1986). Discourse performance in older adults. *International Journal of Aging and Human Development, 23*, 267–283.

Obler, L., & Albert, M. K. (1980). Narrative discourse style in the elderly. In L. K. Obler & M. Albert (Eds.), *Language and communication in the elderly*. Lexington, MA: D.C. Heath.

Obler, L., & Albert, M. L. (1984). Language in aging. In M. L. Albert (Ed.), *Neurology of aging*. New York: Oxford.

Obler, L., Au, R., & Albert, M. L. (in press). Language and aging. In R. Huntley & K. Helfer (Eds.), *Communication and aging*. Andover, MA: Andover Medical.

Tocco, M. (1990, April). *Discourse and aging*. Paper presented at the conference of the New York State Speech, Language and Hearing Association at Kiamesha Lake, NY.

Ulatowska, H., Cannito, M., Hayashi, M., & Fleming, S. (1985). Language abilities in the elderly. In H. Ulatowska (Ed.), *The aging brain: Communication in the elderly* (pp. 125–139). San Diego: College-Hill Press.

Ulatowska, H., Hayashi, M., Cannito, M., & Fleming, S. (1986). Disruption of reference in aging. *Brain and Language, 28*, 24–41.

Chapter 3

Discourse Macrostructure in Aphasia

Hanna K. Ulatowska
Sandra B. Chapman
University of Texas at Dallas

The investigation of discourse ability in aphasia is one of the richest areas in neuropsychology and neurolinguistics in revealing the complex relations that exist between language and cognition. This is so because discourse formulation is an intellectual activity that entails not only the understanding and manipulation of linguistic information, but also involves cognitive operations essential to the organization of information. Despite the abundance of empirical facts that characterize discourse in aphasic patients, relatively little is known regarding what abilities are absolutely necessary for discourse production. In regard to language, the primary issues are: What are the basic linguistic abilities necessary for producing discourse? How do the linguistic prerequisites vary depending on the discourse genre and the conceptual complexity of the discourse text or task? In regard to cognitive ability, the primary issue is: What role does the ability to organize information play in producing well-formed discourse, both as a function of the discourse genre and of the conceptual complexity of the text or task?

The view that grammatically correct sentences do not ensure well-formed discourse and that grammatically incorrect sentences do not necessarily preclude successful discourse production has been upheld across numerous studies (Freedman-Stern, Ulatowska, Baker, & DeLacoste, 1984; Ulatowska & Sadowska, 1992). Indeed, aphasic language patterns are a testimony to this tenet. For example, nonfluent aphasics produce most discourse types in very simple, telegraphic language. This achievement is likely accomplished through a reliance on a more intact ability to structure the information. On the other hand, some patients with relatively preserved language exhibit difficulties in structuring information, thus interfering with discourse ability. This latter discourse has been described as characteristic of the language of patients with Alzheimer's dementia (Chapman & Ulatowska, 1992a; Ulatowska & Chapman, 1991).

This paradoxical disparity between lower levels of language (i.e., lexical and syntactic) and well-formed discourse may be explained, in part, by preservation of macrostructure. Macrostructure refers to the global meaning of texts and is expressed through notions such as theme, topic, gist, and main point (van Dijk, 1980). Well-formed discourse may be guided by an intact macrostructure that allows aphasic patients to produce the central meaning of discourse even with impoverished language. Thus, it is important to consider the contribution of macrostructure when building a model of discourse production (van Dijk, 1980).

With this viewpoint in mind, the goals in this chapter are threefold. The first goal is to define the construct of macrostructure and outline examples of tasks that evaluate aspects of macrostructure. The second is to review the literature relevant to macrostructure in aphasia. The third goal is to illustrate two major issues that need consideration to clarify what impairs the ability of aphasic patients to manipulate macrostructure using four aphasic patients.

The primary issue addressed here is how cognitive and linguistic deficits may be manifested on tasks of macrostructure. Although the separation of cognitive and linguistic factors is artificial, it is important to attempt to unravel the role of each in order to develop appropriate intervention protocols for aphasic patients. The second issue is the contribution of linguistic deficits associated with lesion focus to impairments of macrostructure in discourse. Examination of this latter issue will contribute to the understanding of this relationship across sentential and discourse levels of language. Once the linguistic structures most important for supporting discourse are known, one can target those structures that directly enhance communicative competence in aphasia as therapy goals.

CONSTRUCT OF MACROSTRUCTURE

Definition of Macrostructure

Macrostructures are usually characterized as cognitive structures because they are primarily considered organizational devices of meaning. That is, the macrostructure of a discourse organizes all the propositions of the microlevel text at a higher level of semantic meaning (van Dijk, 1980). The macrostructure operates to facilitate the understanding, organization, and reduction of complex information. Thus, the construct of macrostructure should be accounted for in a cognitive model dealing with recall and comprehension of discourse.

The expression or manipulation of macrostructure has not only a cognitive reality but also a linguistic reality. The cognitive reality of macrostructure is realized through the cognitive operations involved in condensing the information so that the central meaning of a discourse is preserved. This selective reduction is accomplished through retention of the more important information and omission of the less important details (van Dijk, 1980).

This process is not simply one of information reduction, but also of abstracting the information through integration of information to a higher level of generalization. To account for these processes of reduction, Kintsch and van Dijk (1978) delineated three macrorules that operate on a text to selectively reduce the information. These macrorules include the processes of deletion, generalization, and construction. Whereas deletion involves a simple omission of less important information, the processes of generalization and construction replace specific text information with more general or global facts. Whereas macrostructures are often only inferred from a discourse, they are also directly expressed in discourse (i.e., in titles, topic sentences, gists, and summaries).

The linguistic reality of macrostructure is evidenced by the complex linguistic forms required to signal the macrostructure in discourse. The linguistic signaling is referred to as *textual macrostructures*. The textual macrostructures are often more evident in planned, written discourse and are signaled by pronouns, connectives, adverbs, word order, and so on. For example, there are a number of topic change markers at the beginning of new episodes. These markers of topic change include: change of time or period of action, change of place, introduction of new participants, full noun phrase reintroduction of old participants, and change of perspective or point of view indicated by the verb forms.

Superstructure is a related, but not synonymous, construct to macrostructure. The semantic macrostructures require established canonical form of superstructures that are used for developing and organizing a specific discourse genre. For example, the narrative schema is expressed through a temporal sequence of events with a build up of action. This same schema would not be adequate for expository discourse when personal opinions on a particular issue are expressed.

Tasks of Macrostructure

The construct of macrostructure is relatively new and has been investigated only recently in neurolinguistic studies of discourse. However, similar notions have been investigated previously from other perspectives. There is a large body of work by Luria (1980, 1982) that points to the importance of using tasks of macrostructure to assess intellectual abilities in patients with brain lesions. Although Luria did not use the term *macrostructure,* many of the tasks described in his writings tap the global semantic meaning of a text. The stimuli were stories and thematic pictures with probes asking the patients to derive a theme, provide a gist, sequence a series of thematically related pictures and formulate the unifying theme (as opposed to describing each picture separately). Luria also suggested tasks that required the patient to identify the important (essential) details in a text, to synthesize this information, and to reach an interpretation of the global theme. To a large degree, the nature of these tasks involved sorting the information according to importance. This process is critical to understanding the central meaning of a text.

Since the pioneering work by Luria, there have been several investigations utilizing tasks of macrostructure. Siklaki (1984) described a telegram task where the subjects were asked to leave out as much as possible of the original story while trying to retain as much of the important information as possible. Other ways of tapping macrostructure include generating the central event, providing a summary, and even retelling a story. In many instances, the central event conveys the global meaning of the story. In order to produce a summary, it is necessary to abstract what is relevant or essential to the central meaning of the story. The sequence of events in retelling the story also reflects the macrostructure in that the events must follow a logical sequence based on world knowledge and textual knowledge.

All of the macrostructure tasks described here place heavy demands on the language system. In order to explore the contribution of cognitive factors in manipulating macrostructure, some investigators have designed tasks of macrostructure that reduce the linguistic demands. These tasks involved the manipulation of pictures or responses to probes that required minimal verbalization (Huber, 1990; Pierce & Grogan, 1992; Ulatowska & Chapman, 1991). Tasks that assess the ability to logically sequence pictures measure a cognitive aspect of macrostructure without use of verbal language. The ability to remove redundant pictures (i.e., pictures optional to the main storyline) also places greater demand on the cognitive system than the linguistic (Ulatowska & Chapman, 1991).

In addition to sequencing pictures and removing unimportant pictures within a sequence, probe questions have been utilized to evaluate cognitive aspects of macrostructure. The questions were structured so that the language requirements were minimized. These structured probe questions involved identifying the main props or characters, responding to sentence completions, answering multiple-choice questions and answering questions relevant to setting information (Pierce & Grogan, 1992; Ulatowska & Chapman, 1991).

What is to be gleaned from the discussion here is a sense of how macrostructure in neurolinguistic research can be studied. Specifically, various tasks that tap macrostructure are outlined; however, this list of tasks is in no way exhaustive. Two major points regarding the nature of macrostructure should be made. First, tasks that manipulate macrostructure require that information from the original stimulus be transformed or reconstructed in discourse production. This transformation involves a reduction of information while preserving the central meaning. In the process of transforming or restructuring the text, the information is not simply deleted; but, rather it is constructed and generalized to an abstract level. The second point is that intactness of macrostructure may need to be examined utilizing tasks with varying demands on the cognitive and linguistic systems.

MACROSTRUCTURE IN APHASIA

The documentation of preserved information structure in aphasic discourse despite marked difficulties in sentential abilities has been validated in a number of studies (Dressler & Pleh, 1988; Glosser & Deser, 1991; Huber, 1990; Ulatowska & Chapman, 1991; Ulatowska, Freedman-Stern, Doyel, Macaluso-Haynes, & North, 1983; Ulatowska, North, & Macaluso-Haynes, 1981). The claim that discourse is preserved relative to sentential abilities does not preclude a relationship between lower levels (word and sentence) and higher levels (discourse) of language (Caplan, 1992). Nor does this claim necessarily imply that discourse processing is unimpaired in aphasia (Chapman & Ulatowska, 1992b; Huber, 1990). Indeed, certain studies have reported disturbances of macrostructure in aphasia (Chapman & Ulatowska, 1992; Pierce & Grogan, 1992; Ulatowska & Sadowska, 1992; Ulatowska, Sadowska, Kordys, & Kadzielawa, in press). The disturbances appear as a result of differences in the quantity of information, the distribution of information, the level of generalization for responses, and the way macrostructure information is signaled in the language system. These disturbances are manifested by disruption in the application of the macrorules (i.e., deletion, construction, and generalization—described earlier).

Manipulation of Macrorules

The application of the macrorules of deletion, construction, and generalization performs the function of producing the appropriate amount and quality of information. The rule of deletion controls the amount of information in that it does not allow for the inclusion of redundant or unnecessary information. The rules of construction and especially generalization are responsible for the abstraction of information at an appropriate level.

Quantity of Information. There is a convergence of evidence that aphasic patients show a reduction of information in discourse (Berko Gleason et al., 1980; Ulatowska et al., 1981, 1983). This reduction of information was selective in that the most important information was recalled, whereas the less important details were omitted from the retellings. Initially, this selective reduction of information was interpreted to mean that narrative structure was relatively well preserved in aphasia. However, this interpretation has been modified recently in light of evidence from subsequent studies. The early evidence related to preservation of superstructure in aphasic discourse production rather than macrostructure. Ulatowska and Sadowska (1992) claimed that superstructure replaced macrostructure in guiding aphasic patients' discourse, where superstructure defined the structure and macrostructure referred to the global semantic meaning of discourse (van Dijk & Kintsch, 1983).

The reduction of information disrupts macrostructure (even in simple narratives) by interfering with story development in aphasic patients' narratives. When information is reduced to a simple concatenation of facts as is common in aphasic discourse, the resultant narratives lack the appropriate build up to the climax or turning point of the story (Ulatowska et al., 1983). In contrast, there is a gradual build up of action signaling the turning point of the story in normal subjects. This aspect of signaling the climax of a story is important to macrostructure.

In aphasic patients the impact of reduced information on macrostructure is more apparent in spontaneous discourse productions and in more complex narratives (e.g., increased number of episodes) as compared to retold information using simple narratives (Ulatowska & Sadowska, 1992). For simple narrative retellings, there may not be enough information to reveal aphasic patients' difficulties with macrostructure.

Distribution of Information. Macrostructure can also be impaired as a result of a skewed distribution of information within the individual story components (e.g., setting, action, and resolution). Evidence has shown that setting information in the narrative discourse of aphasic patients is increased as compared to the amount of information given in the other story components (Ulatowska et al., 1981; Ulatowska et al., 1983; Ulatowska & Sadowska, 1992). Setting information may be more resistant to disruption because this type of information is easier to express, cognitively and linguistically. The setting usually specifies the participants, the place, and the time of the story. Normally, the setting is stated as a simple listing of the pieces of information. The linguistic form of the information contained in the setting is expressed as a set of simple sentences primarily with stative verbs. The conceptual and linguistic simplicity of the setting information is contrasted to the complexity that typically characterizes the event sequence of the story.

Further support for the impaired distribution of information in aphasic discourse is reflected in the evidence that aphasic patients produce too much detail in summaries (Ulatowska et al., 1983; Ulatowska, Allard, & Chapman, 1990; Ulatowska & Chapman, 1991). This inappropriate amount of detail in summaries suggests that many aphasic patients may not be able to manipulate the macrorules as required to reduce complex information in order to preserve the macrostructure.

Studies of aphasic discourse have suggested that macrostructure may be impaired by an inappropriate balance between explicit and implicit information. Even in retellings, there is evidence that some aphasic patients produce excessive detail in trying to relay the story (Ulatowska & Sadowska, 1992). This excessive detail may result from an impaired sensitivity to what information needs to be made explicit and what information can be implied.

Level of Generalization. Many aphasic patients give responses that are bound to the explicit textual information producing a type of concrete response even when the task requires a more generalized response (Chapman & Ulatowska, 1992b;

Ulatowska et al., in press). The concrete response strategy common to aphasics may be a manifestation of an inappropriate application of the macrorules. Aphasic patients may have difficulty conveying the global gist of the message if the response involves combining world knowledge and textual knowledge. In extremely difficult processing conditions, aphasics often rely primarily on world knowledge that in some cases may be inappropriate and may lead to failure (Huber, 1990).

Linguistic Signaling of Information

Another feature of aphasic discourse that disrupts macrostructure relates to how old and new information are signaled linguistically. Aphasic patients have difficulty marking old and new information is evidenced in referential marking and signaling backgrounded information through embedding. In regard to referential marking, Ulatowska and Sadowska (1992) showed how macrostructure is impaired in a mild aphasic patient through the signaling of referents. This patient introduced actors with specific terms instead of the normal pattern of general terms on the first mention.

In order to produce macrostructure, it is imperative that some information is backgrounded and/or embedded whereas other information is foregrounded. Aphasic patients have difficulty embedding information and often produce all of the information at the same level (Caplan, 1992; Ulatowska et al., 1983; Ulatowska & Sadowska, 1992). This problem may be a consequence of disruption of the linguistic system because certain syntactic structures (dependent clauses, adverbial phrases at episode boundaries, topic sentences, and summary paragraphs) that are needed to signal different levels of information may be impaired in aphasia (Ulatowska & Sadowska, 1992).

EXEMPLIFICATION OF MACROSTRUCTURE IN APHASIC DISCOURSE

In this section, the performance of four aphasic patients is illustrated using various tasks that manipulate macrostructure. These particular patients were selected to illustrate two points. One point is that macrostructure may be impaired as a result of cognitive deficits, linguistic deficits, or a combination of both. The performances of the first two patients on the various discourse tasks illustrate how macrostructure disruption may be reflective of impairment in abstract attitude (as in the case of Patient 1) or of impairment in language (Patient 2). The second point is that the linguistic characteristics related to lesion locus may be important to consider in order to elucidate mechanisms contributing to patients' difficulties in manipulating macrostructure. Aphasic Patient 3 and Patient 4 manifested two different types of aphasia, anterior and posterior aphasias, respectively. Whereas differences in lesion location have been associated with different disruptions at a sentential level, the impact on discourse of the differential language breakdown according to lesion locus is not clear.

Issue 1: Is the Impairment of Macrostructure Due to Cognitive or Linguistic Factors?

The stimuli used to tap macrostructure for Patients 1 and 2 were selected Aesop's fables. The specific macrostructure tasks of interest in this chapter include providing the main idea/gist and the moral for the story. These two tasks represent a subset of macrostructure tasks that are part of a larger study and that has been described elsewhere (Chapman & Ulatowska, 1992b; Ulatowska et al., in press). The tasks of gist and moral were selected for illustrative purposes because they appear to be the most revealing in terms of elucidating underlying mechanisms of impaired macrostructure. This may be due to the cognitive complexity of these two tasks because they involve a generalized response to a broader context than the textual information.

The stimuli used to elicit the gist and the moral were three Aesop's fables and one fablelike picture sequence story. The stimuli had a length of 12 to 15 propositions and were written in simple language. The content of the fables evolved around a trick used by the protagonist to achieve his goal. The trick is exemplified by the fox using flattery to steal cheese from the raven (*Raven and Fox*) and by the fox tricking the dog into wrapping his leash around the tree so the fox could steal the dog's meat (*Dog and Fox* picture-sequence story). Conceptual complexity of the stimuli was introduced in a fable where the "trick" was not successful. Such was the case in the fable of the raven who painted his feathers white in order to disguise himself as a pigeon in order to eat the pigeons' food; but in the end, the raven was chased away by the pigeons as well as by his own kind when he tried to return to them (*Raven and Pigeons*). Additional complexity was also represented in a fable where the meaning of the story had to be derived from the interpretation of the metaphoric use of language. In this fable (*Old Woman and Doctor*), the doctor's scheme of stealing his patient's (the old woman's) belongings is unveiled by a clever play on words by the old woman.

Patient 1. Patient 1 is a 52-year-old man with 2 years of college education. He suffered a single cerebral vascular accident approximately 8 years ago. At the time of testing his language had recovered to a relatively high level as suggested by a severity rating of 4 (out of 5) on the Boston Diagnostic Aphasia Examination (BDAE). A severity rating of 4 indicates that the patient had some obvious loss of fluency but not to the extent that the expression of ideas was significantly limited (Goodglass & Kaplan, 1983). For exemplification purposes, the patient's responses are indicated below for the four stimuli described earlier.

Fox and Dog

Gist: The dog is supposed to run around the tree and the fox gets the meat.

Moral: Don't go around and round a tree and with a leash on or a fox is gonna get your meat.

Raven and Fox

Gist: Don't open your mouth if you have cheese.

Moral: If you're raven, don't open your mouth if you have cheese.

Old Woman and Doctor

Gist: She could see her belongings before he came but she could not see them afterwards.

Moral: If the doctor is stealing, get him right quick.

Raven and Pigeons

Gist: Stay like you are and don't paint your feathers.

Moral: Don't paint your feathers.

The most prominent feature of Patient 1's discourse was the generation of texts using information contained within the original text. The patient's responses were derived primarily from textual information and are referred to as *intratextual* responses. Notice that all of Patient 1's responses for gist and moral adhere closely to the original text for all four stories. In contrast, normal individuals typically produce responses that generalize to the world at large, particularly for moral probes and to a large degree, even for gist probes using fables (Ulatowska et al., in press). Responses that integrate textual information with world knowledge are referred to as *extratextual* responses.

The tendency toward producing intratextual responses was consistent across all probes for all stories for Patient 1. The patient's responses showed minimal departure from the original text, despite the fact that the probes required a generalized response beyond the specific content of the story. Even with further questioning from the examiner directing the patient to apply the moral of the fable to people's lives, the patient was not able to shift from the specific story content.

Several explanations may be offered for the patient's performance. One explanation for the patient's reluctance to depart from the original text may be a failure to understand the task. However, he seemed to understand the task of providing a lesson/moral as evidenced by his production of speech acts of admonition or warning using the imperative form. Another explanation for his difficulties on macrostructure tasks that require generalizing beyond the explicit story content might be linguistic difficulties. Whereas language impairment may contribute in some degree to this patient's problems in producing generalized responses, this explanation seems inadequate for two reasons. One reason is that the patient exhibits relatively complex language as exemplified by the use of multiple embedded clauses within sentential units (see moral response for *Raven and Fox* and gist response for *Old Woman and Doctor*). The second reason is the evidence that normal subjects produce generalized responses with simple language.

We suggest that the primary factor contributing to the patient's difficulties is the impairment of abstract attitude. The concept of abstract attitude to describe this patient's verbal responses is not ideal because it is broad and multifaceted (Benton, 1991); however, the term captures the essence of this patient's tendency toward production of concrete responses, shown by an impairment in the ability to generalize. Patient 1's responses are bound to the information expressed in the stimulus text. Further support for this postulation is his performance on a separate task involving proverbs (Delis, Kramer, & Kaplan, 1984). Proverbs have been utilized for many years to evaluate verbal abstraction ability. Interpreting proverbs accurately requires an intact fund of general information and the ability to apply this knowledge to a broader context than the specific content (Strub & Black, 1985). Patient 1 did not go beyond the specific text of the individual proverbs either on spontaneous explanations of the proverb meaning or on a multiple choice task (given four choices for the proverb's meaning). The following two response choices reflect his reluctance to go beyond the specific content. For the proverb: "Too many cooks spoil the broth," his response choice was: "One person can make soup better than 10." The correct response was: "A task is at risk when more people are involved than are needed." For the proverb: "Don't count your chickens before they are hatched," his response choice was: "There may be fewer chicks than there were eggs," instead of the more appropriate response: "One shouldn't always assume that things will turn out the way one expects."

Patient 2. Patient 2 exhibited greater impairment of language than Patient 1, as evidenced by the responses that follow here, and by his severity rating of 2.5 on the BDAE. Patient 2 was a 44-year-old man with 3 years of college education at the time of testing. He suffered a single cerebral vascular accident approximately 7 years prior to testing. Until then, he had been working as a plant manager in his own business. His responses on the four fables follow.

Fox and Dog

Gist: Thinking . . . thinking right here, by brain thinking.

Moral: Well . . . it's . . . fox is smart . . . OK, and then a dog is uh, a dog is not so smart.

Fox and Raven

Gist: Well . . . well . . . the same thing is s-smart everything, uh smart . . . and the brain, OK.

Moral: A raven, raven is dumb, OK, fox smart, very smart . . . raven is not . . . yeah..

Old Woman and Doctor

Gist: Doctor is set, money, money, money . . . no for . . . no it's, doctor is it, take it all but . . . it's hard for me . . . it's doctor, money, money, money.

Moral: Watch out money.

Raven and Pigeons

Gist: Body is the same, body is just right just like that and turn it around, it's wrong.

Moral: Body is fine, OK, but paint is no good, you see. You're fine, OK, but change it . . . it's bad.

The most prominent feature of Patient 2's discourse is his dramatic struggle in trying to find the words to convey the meaning for the gist and moral probes. This patient adopts a simplistic strategy of evaluating the characters in the fables in terms of antonymous dichotomies. For example, he contrasts the fox as "smart" and the dog as "not smart" in the *Fox and Dog* story. Similarly, he characterizes the fox as "smart" and the raven as "dumb" in the *Fox and Raven* fable. In the *Raven and Pigeons*, he tries to get the meaning across with the contrastive terms *right* and *wrong*. Even in this simplistic strategy, Patient 2's responses are of an inferential nature although they are still derived primarily from the content of the stimulus fable.

For Patient 2, it is clearly his language impairment that is the primary obstruction to his ability to produce abstract responses. This is not to say that cognitive factors are not a contributing factor, but their role seems secondary to the linguistic factors.

This presumption of the primary role of linguistic factors in his difficulties of producing abstract responses is supported by his performance on the Proverb Test. Patient 2's linguistic difficulties were pervasive in his attempts to spontaneously explain the meaning of the proverbs. However, in contrast to Patient 1, Patient 2's responses on the multiple-choice task were the appropriate abstract meaning in that the interpretation generalized to a broader context than the specific proverb content. He gave correct abstract responses to all 10 proverbs.

In summary, the responses of Patient 1 and Patient 2 show that both cognitive and linguistic factors can disrupt the ability to manipulate macrostructure. For Patient 1, the difficulties in transforming texts on tasks of macrostructure were due more to cognitive factors than linguistic factors as reflected in his inability to generalize. Patient 2, on the other hand, was limited primarily by his linguistic deficits. As more is learned about the mechanisms contributing to impairment of macrostructure, the information should be useful clinically, both in diagnostics and rehabilitation.

Issue 2: Do Linguistic Abilities Associated With Lesion Site Contribute to Impairment of Macrostructure?

The main focus of these latter two case presentations is to illustrate how certain language impairments may contribute to disruption of macrostructure. Specifically, the impact of impaired language features important for signaling macro- and microstructure are discussed in relation to different aphasic language profiles derived from anterior and posterior lesions in two mildly impaired aphasic patients.

The stimuli used to evaluate macrostructure for Patients 3 and 4 involved spontaneously produced narrative and expository discourse as well as retelling of fables with the same probes described for Patients 1 and 2. The patients' discourses were written with unlimited time constraints. These two patients were part of a larger study conducted in Poland and are described elsewhere (Ulatowska & Sadowska, 1992). Whereas the task of retelling fables provided a specific macrostructure to guide discourse production, the macrostructure was not given in spontaneous discourse productions. Thus, the patients had more freedom to choose any possible way of producing macrostructure, instead of simply reconstructing it from the stimulus given.

The difference in content across discourse genres places different requirements on the linguistic system in terms of the complex structures required to support and signal macrostructure. The different linguistic requirements are due to the fact that the complexity of macrostructure is affected by characteristics of the content. For example, narrative discourse is characterized by a highly conventional structure involving a sequence of events. In contrast, expository discourse has a variety of possible structures that can be selected to suit one's own preferences and cognitive style. Narrative macrostructure can be achieved by a simple concatenation of propositions with a strong temporal organization. Expository discourse, on the other hand, lacks this type of structure and requires more complex syntactic marking of information.

Patient 3. Patient 3 presented with an anterior aphasia after suffering a stroke at 36 years of age. He recovered to a relatively mild aphasia as indicated by a severity rating of 4 on the BDAE. Prior to his stroke, he was a patent lawyer.

This patient exhibited impairment of macrostructure as signaled by a disruption of the information structure and/or as reflected by disruptions at a linguistic level. In regard to information structure, Patient 3 showed a reduction of macrostructure types in that most of his discourse productions were reduced to descriptive and narrative types. This preference for a specific content type occurred even when eliciting other genres (e.g., expository). Additionally, Patient 3 exhibited disruption of macrostructure at an information structure level as reflected by an inappropriate distribution of information. The inclusion of too many details resulted in "overspecificity" that was characteristic of his discourse. He seemed insensitive as to what information should be explicit and what should be implicit. This tendency of overspecificity was also evident in his difficulties to summarize as he included main ideas as well as less important information in his summaries. In regard to language, it is important to note that he showed an overall reduction in complexity of language consistent with the "classic characteristics" of aphasic patients with anterior lesions. He also showed difficulties in marking reference in the way old and new information are signaled in that he primarily used nouns with only a limited use of pronouns.

In order to examine Patient 3's performance on more structured tasks of macrostructure, his responses are provided for the gist and moral tasks of macrostructure using the four fables.

Raven and Pigeons
Gist: Certain environment and food
Moral: The raven painted his feathers white and crowed. Other kinds and the raven kind did not accept him.

The Old Woman and Doctor
Gist: The court ruled in favor of the old woman.
Moral: The old woman said that her sight deteriorated. The court agreed with her argument and ruled in her favor. The court thought that the law is on the old woman's side.

Raven and Fox
Gist: It concerns the fox and raven who held a piece of cheese in his beak. The cheese fell on the ground. The raven grabbed it.
Moral: The fox decided to get the food by any means and he got it.

As indicated by these responses, Patient 3 exhibited a consistent pattern of concrete, intratextual responses. The intratextual responses confirm the rigidity and preference for a narrative type content as observed by his spontaneously produced discourse on a variety of topics. His responses also show the same difficulty in reducing information. In a way, his tendency to give summaries on the moral probe show a similar pattern of overspecificity as noted in his spontaneous discourse.

Patient 4. Patient 4 presented with a posterior aphasia that had recovered to a mild level of aphasia as indicated by a severity rating of 4 on the BDAE. This patient had a stroke at age 39 and was a psychologist prior to the stroke. The patient was seen for evaluation and experimental discourse therapy approximately 2 years after the stroke.

Patient 4 was able to manipulate macrostructure successfully on a number of tasks as well as in a variety of discourse genres varying in complexity. She used topic sentences and summary paragraphs as transitions between topics or types of information. She successfully embedded different types of discourse within each other (e.g., embedding of narrative and expository genres within conversation).

Disturbances of macrostructure were observed in Patient 4's discourse primarily at the level of signaling macrostructure. Her discourse lacked anaphoric and transition connectors between different topics of information. She also had difficulty manipulating terms of reference that impaired macrostructure. For example, she started with more specific referential terms and then later used less specific terms, contrary to normal patterns of referential marking. She did not always mark aspect or tense of verbs that disrupted the flow of information. Finally, she had problems signaling old and new information. New information is typically foregrounded in independent clauses and old information is backgrounded in dependent clauses. On occasion, this patient used a reverse pattern with old information expressed through independent clauses that caused a disruption of focus in macrostructure.

In contrast to Patient 3's intratextual responses on the fable tasks, Patient 4 gave generalized, extratextual responses. This patient was able to summarize, to provide gists, and to generate morals as shown on her responses below. Her responses on these fable tasks confirmed her observed success in combining different types of information. However, it is important to note that her difficulty with linguistic marking of macrostructure was not revealed on the fable tasks. The insensitivity of fable probes to identify her linguistic deficits in marking macrostructure is probably due to her high language ability and to the nature of the tasks (i.e., gist and moral require relatively brief responses).

Raven and Fox
Gist: Compliments are not always true.
Moral: The moral is clear—if one looks after one's own belongings, one has them, if not, he does not have them.

Raven and Pigeons
Gist: It does not pay to change one's appearance.
Moral: It applies not only to color but to people who want to change their country or their social group in communist Poland.

The Old Woman and Doctor
Gist: Everyone senses things in one's own house.
Moral: One should not deceive an old person. The old woman was not defeated by her sickness and did not lose her sense of humor.

In summary, the language performances of Patient 3 and Patient 4 indicated that the different language profiles for anterior versus posterior aphasic patients can affect the ability to signal certain aspects of macrostructure, linguistically. The comparison of these two patients also revealed that the complexity of schemata necessary for the production of some discourse genres (e.g., expository) may be restricted by certain types of aphasia.

CONCLUSION

In conclusion, the investigation of macrostructure in aphasic discourse is important for theoretical and clinical reasons. The theoretical importance of studying macrostructure lies in its value of illuminating the nature of the complex relationship between cognitive and linguistic aspects in the production and comprehension of discourse. The study of macrostructure clarifies how information structure can facilitate language and how language can serve as an important vehicle through which information structure is carried.

The clinical importance of macrostructure lies in its potential value in defining communicative competence of speakers in terms of coherence (organizational structure) and cohesion (its linguistic form). The study of macrostructure may also elucidate the relationship between coherence and cohesion. Moreover, the information derived from studies of macrostructure may contribute to the process of making a differential diagnosis. Different patient groups (e.g., focal lesions versus diffuse lesions, or right- versus left-hemispheric lesioned patients), may eventually be differentiated neurolinguistically by patterns of disruptions and preservations, not only in the operations of linguistic rules of syntax and semantics but also in the operation of macrorules in specific communicative contexts.

Finally, a macrostructure approach to therapy may be particularly beneficial to patients. The approach will vary depending on a number of factors including whether the deficits appear to be more conceptual or linguistic and the severity of the impairment.

If a patient's problem in manipulating information structure is more conceptual, the patient may benefit by exposure to a variety of tasks with different types of information structure. Tasks could be varied along a range of conceptual complexity, from the simplest to the most complex. For example, the simplest information structure is manifested in stories for which all the information necessary for understanding the deep meaning of the text is explicitly stated. Increasing the complexity can be achieved by using stories that contain implicit information. Implicit information requires more inferencing in order to understand the deep meaning.

Some other ways to help patients with conceptual difficulties in manipulating information may be achieved by presenting information in different modalities (e.g., pictorial vs. verbal representation). The different modes of presentation make certain relationships more salient and easier to understand.

Improving patients' ability to manipulate information structure should be approached by systematically building a natural progression of complexity into the tasks. For example, in the approach described for the case studies, the information needed to identify and provide justification for the main character is probed before the gist information because it is conceptually simple. Another dimension related to progression is the interdependence of meaning that exists among different types of information. For example, it is not possible to appreciate the moral of a fable unless the main character is appropriately identified. This interdependence should be taken into account in sequencing tasks of information structure.

Another technique to help patients with conceptual difficulties is to use tasks with multiple-choice responses. These tasks can be used to help the patient select generalized responses that utilize extratextual information. At a higher level of complexity, information structure can be manipulated by having patients identify similarities and differences between fables with similar morals. At the highest level, different discourse genres can be manipulated to increase the conceptual complexity. For example, expository discourse is characterized by more complex information structure than either narrative or procedural discourse.

Different approaches have to be adopted with patients for whom the primary problem is language difficulties in marking the micro- and macrostructure. These difficulties typically affect two types of cohesive ties (i.e., marking reference and providing transitional links between micro- and macrostructures). At this level, techniques to help patients with their language problems can involve analytical tasks of a metalinguistic nature. For example, patients can be asked to identify all the terms used to signal the characters/props throughout a story. This task makes the patient aware of instances when specific references (e.g., nouns) should be used as opposed to nonspecific referents (i.e., pronouns), for example at the beginning of new episodes. Potential ambiguities of reference occur when the referential terms are not used properly. Another task that manipulates the marking of reference is to provide stories where referential slots are left empty. Then, the patient is requested to fill the slots with nouns or pronouns.

A similar technique can be used to build transitions using appropriate connectors between macrostructures. Patients can be asked to identify points where certain links are needed. Then specific connectors such as *then, so, finally* are provided by the clinician. To increase the complexity of the task, stories can be given where the patient has to supply the link. It should be stressed that these metalinguistic tasks are suitable primarily for patients with mild to moderate language problems and with relatively good abilities to structure information in the stories. With more severely impaired patients, intervention approaches of facilitating phrasal and sentential structures could be employed with the emphasis on rebuilding verb structures since verbs provide the backbone of any discourse.

In summary, we suggest that a macrostructure approach may be more relevant and efficacious than more traditional approaches. This type approach may help to improve the patients' communicative strategies and not only their linguistic structures.

ACKNOWLEDGMENTS

This research was supported by a grant from the Texas Advanced Research Program (#009741-013), by grant AG 09486-01A1 from the National Institute on Aging, and by a grant from the National Academy of Sciences.

REFERENCES

Benton, A. L. (1991). The prefrontal region: Its early history. In H. S. Levin, H. M. Eisenberg, & A. L. Benton (Eds.), *Frontal lobe function and dysfunction* (pp. 3–34). New York: Oxford University Press.

Berko Gleason, G., Goodglass, H., Obler, L.., Green, E., Hyde, M., & Weintraub, S. (1980). Narrative strategies of aphasic and normal speaking subjects. *Journal of Speech and Hearing Research, 23*, 370–382.

Caplan, D. (1992). *Language: Structure, processing and disorders*. Cambridge, MA: MIT Press.

Chapman, S. B., & Ulatowska, H. K. (1992a). Methodology for discourse management in the treatment of aphasia. *Clinics in Communication Disorders, 2*(1), 64–81.

Chapman, S. B., & Ulatowska, H. K. (1992b). The nature of language disruption in dementia: Is it aphasia? *Texas Journal of Audiology and Speech Pathology*, 3–9.

Delis, D., Kramer, J., & Kaplan, E. (1984). *The California proverb test*. Unpublished protocol.

Dressler, W. U., & Pleh, C. (1988). On text disturbances in aphasia. In W. U. Dressler & J. A. Stark (Eds.), *Linguistic analyses of aphasic language* (pp. 151–178). New York: Springer-Verlag.

Freedman-Stern, R., Ulatowska, H. K., Baker, T., & DeLacoste, C. (1984). Disruption of written language in aphasia: A case study. *Brain and Language, 21*, 181–205.

Glosser, G., & Deser, T. (1991). Patterns of discourse production among neurological patients with fluent language disorders. *Brain and Language, 40*, 67–88.

Goodglass, H., & Kaplan, E. (1983). *The assessment of aphasia and related disorders* (2nd ed.). Philadelphia: Lea & Febiger.

Huber, W. (1990). Text comprehension and production in aphasia: Analysis in terms of micro- and macrostructure. In Y. Joanette & H. H. Brownell (Eds.), *Discourse ability and brain damage: Theoretical and empirical perspectives* (pp. 154–179). New York: Springer-Verlag.

Kintsch, W., & van Dijk, T. A. (1978). Toward a model of text comprehension and production. *Psychological Review, 85*, 363–394.

Luria, A. R. (1980). *Higher cortical functions in man* (2nd ed.). New York: Basic Books.

Luria, A. R. (1982). *Language and cognition*. Washington, DC: V. H. Winston.

Pierce, R. S., & Grogan, S. (1992). Improving listening comprehension of narratives. *Clinics in Communication Disorders, 2*, 54–63.

Siklaki, I. (1984). Macro-structure, knowledge base, and coherence. *Text and Discourse Connectedness, 16*, 309–324.

Strub, R. L., & Black, F. W. (1985). *The mental status examination in neurology*. Philadelphia: F. A. Davis.

Ulatowska, H. K., Allard, L., & Chapman, S. B. (1990). Narrative and procedural discourse in aphasia. In Y. Joanette & H. H. Brownell (Eds.), *Discourse ability and brain damage: Theoretical and empirical perspectives*. New York: Springer-Verlag.

Ulatowska, H. K., & Chapman, S. B. (1991). Language and studies and dementia. In R. Lubinski (Ed.), *Dementia in communication: Research and clinical implications*. Philadelphia: B. C. Decker.

Ulatowska, H. K., Freedman-Stern, R., Doyel, A. W., Macaluso-Haynes, S., & North, A. J. (1983). Production of narrative discourse in aphasia. *Brain and Language, 19*, 317–334.

Ulatowska, H. K., North, A. J., & Macaluso-Haynes, S. (1981). Production of narrative and procedural discourse in aphasia. *Brain and Language, 13*, 345–371.

Ulatowska, H. K., & Sadowska, M. (1992). Some observations on aphasic texts. In S. J. Hrang & W. R. Merrifield (Eds.), *Language in context: Essays for Robert E. Longacre* (pp. 51–66). Arlington: The Summer Institute of Linguistics and the University of Texas at Arlington.

Ulatowska, H. K., Sadowska, M., Kordys, J., & Kadzielawa, D. (1993). Selected aspects of narratives in Polish speaking aphasics as illustrated by Aesop's fables. In Y. Joanette & H. Brownell (Eds.), *Narrative discourse in normal aging and neurologically impaired adults*. San Diego: Singular Publishing Group.

van Dijk, T. A. (1980). *Macrostructures: An interdisciplinary study of global structures in discourse, interaction and cognition.* Hillsdale, NJ: Lawrence Erlbaum Associates.

van Dijk, T. A., & Kintsch, W. (1983). *Strategies of discourse comprehension.* New York: Academic Press.

Chapter 4

A Method for Microanalysis of Discourse in Brain-Damaged Patients

Anita Haravon
Loraine K. Obler
The City University of New York Graduate School

Martha Taylor Sarno
New York University, School of Medicine

Discourse analysis done with brain-damaged patients has focused on larger units of discourse such as story structure and content elements (Bloom, 1990; Ehrlich, 1990; Ulatowska, Freedman-Sterm, Doyel, Macaluso-Haynes, & North, 1983). Saffran, Berndt, and Schwartz (1989) proposed techniques for analysis of the discourse of agrammatic patients in which they focus on more microlevel constituents. They provide algorithms for determining the number of utterances as well as words and for structural measures such as the number of embeddings, measures of well-formedness, and the syntactic constituents within sentences.

This chapter reports on our attempt to expand Saffran et al.'s analysis for use with all aphasic patients who produce more than minimal amounts of speech and, by extension, for brain-damaged patients who are not frankly aphasic but whose language patterns share some similarities with those of aphasics. The analysis we propose, we suspect, will also be of use for mild to moderately impaired patients with dementia of the Alzheimer type. Elements of our proposed analysis were modified and employed in Ehrlich, Obler, Clark, and Gerstman (1993, and see Ehrlich, chapter 9, this volume) and in Nicholas, Obler, Albert, and Helm-Estabrooks (1985). We structure the chapter as follows: First we sketch the development of the system we propose, noting our emphasis on morphology, lexicon, and phrase-level structures. Then we discuss particulars of our analytical suggestions, referring readers to the handbook that constitutes Appendix A. Appendix B includes samples of the transcriptions and coding of one relatively fluent aphasic patient and Appendix C includes samples of the transcription and coding of one nonfluent patient.

The analytic system we propose evolved for a study of recovery from aphasia as it relates to age,[1] and a study of the discourse changes of normal aging by the second author.[2] Thus, the focus of the microanalysis was to determine the extent to which narrative texture changes over the course of recovery. The system was employed for the first approximately 100 subjects (fluent, nonfluent, and global aphasics) in the recovery from aphasia project and many modifications were required to adapt it for analysis of the aphasics' speech.

As the Cookie Theft Picture from the Boston Diagnostic Aphasia Exam (Goodglass & Kaplan, 1972; see Appendix D) is widely used in aphasia diagnosis, we selected it for our study. Subjects were asked to tell the story of what was going on in the Cookie Theft Picture and the narrative was transcribed. (A single pass through the tape was virtually never sufficient to record all the utterances, consequently numerous passes were made in order to have the most complete transcription possible.) Because responses are relatively short and descriptive, overarching measures of story structure were not crucial (see Ulatowska et al., 1983, for references to these). We did determine the number of themes based on the eight that can be found in the Cookie Theft Picture (mother/woman/lady, washing/wiping/drying/doing dishes, water overflowing out of sink, boy/kids, stealing/reaching for cookies, stool tipping/boy falling off stool, girl/sister, mother not paying attention/oblivious). We also considered whether the patients connected themes in their narratives. The two common themes connected are:

1. The mother doesn't notice that the children are stealing cookies.
2. The mother doesn't notice that the sink is overflowing.

For purposes of the microanalysis, our primary focus was morphological units and lexical types as well as syntactic errors within sentences, and *aposiopesis*, "the abrupt termination of an utterance that leaves a thought incomplete" (Hier, Hagenlocker, & Shindler, 1985, p. 119). We also considered the pragmatic function served by sentences that were not part of the narrative structure (Saffran et al., 1989, by contrast, focus only on the narrative structure).

Note that the system we propose is particularly effective for mild to moderately impaired patients. For patients producing only jargon and/or stereotypies or severely perseverative patients, the coding we propose is less effective. Nevertheless, it can be of use to simply code such patients as unscoreable under one of three categories: jargon plus stereotypies or automatic speech; jargon plus real words (including some meaningful content words); and real word repetition irrelevant to the task (e.g., "fish, fish, fish").

---

[1]This was an NIH study directed by the third author entitled "Age, Linguistic Evolution, and Quality of Life in Aphasia."

[2]This study was conducted in the Language in the Aging Brain Lab of the Boston VA Medical Center.

MORPHOLOGY

Units

Our goal in counting the number of units is to distinguish the units spoken by the subject in performing the narrative test from filler items, jargon items, and stereotypies, and to determine the percentage of the text that repetition and repairs contribute. First a determination of the total number of units was made that included all repetitions, false starts, and fillers. For this count, for example, when the fluent aphasic (Appendix B, line 1) says "There's a a young" we counted five units (contraction is counted as two units). After determining the total number of units, the total number of repetitions, false starts, and repairs was determined.

We find it particularly helpful to use colored pencils in making these analyses so that we have a record of what items were counted under what categories. Different colors as well as different markings (e.g., wavy lines, circles, etc.) help the researcher check classification and counts of items, which is invariably necessary. (See Appendix A for examples of classifications.)

Repetitions were coded as syllable repetitions, word repetitions, and phrase repetitions (see Appendix A, p. 54). False starts can be distinguished from sentence fragments or aposiopesis because what follows a false start is what it was in fact starting, whereas what aposiopesis follows is unrelated. Thus, "/kI/, kitchen" is scored as one repetition or false start. (Also, see Appendix C, p. 72.)

Counts were made on units to the first prompt. For discourse responses greater than 100 words, we conducted an analysis of eight patients, tallying their entire response up to the first prompt and their response just considering the first 100 words and determined that the quality of the discourse does not change markedly. Thus, we recommend using only the first 100 words unless one is collecting rare phenomena such as paragrammatic errors (e.g., in Appendix B only the first 100 words were analyzed).

Word Class

Two overarching categories (substantives and functors) were used, and subcategory analyses were conducted within that dichotomy. Substantives included nouns, verbs (both main and infinitival), gerunds, adjectives, and adverbs. Although it is generally easier to divide words into substantives and functors, adverbs serve as an intermediate category and can be quite problematic. Adverbs ending in "ly" are clearly adjectives, but a number of other adverbs (per dictionary definition) such as "ever," "never," "all," in the phrase "all alone," and the like, appear to have the role of functors and were thus included as such. Similarly, although educated people tend to think that sentences can be easily divided into nouns, verbs, and so on, one finds numerous difficulties in lexical class analysis of text. Some problems arose, for example, with respect to the adjective class.

Nouns that are used as adjectives (e.g., "cookie" in "cookie jar") were considered adjectives for this analysis as they represent a more complex syntactic structure. Also, adjectives of quantity (e.g., "many," "some") were considered functors and thus not included in the adjective count.

Note that dictionaries can be used to help determine part of speech but in the end some instances will remain unclear anyway and one simply has to assure that one is making decisions in a systematic way. For our first pass through the materials we permitted ourselves the opportunity to consider words either clear-cut cases of substantives or functors or questionable cases. In fact, the questionable category was used for jargon terms and was also used for paragrammatic or agrammatic utterances. It was sometimes unclear whether a word that occurs in more than one word class (e.g., "dance") was being employed as a noun or a verb.

With respect to functors, we included pronouns, auxiliary, copula, modal verbs, and conjunctions. We also included a miscellaneous category for articles, prepositions, and other words that shared frequency and length characteristics with functors and do not clearly fall into the substantive category (e.g., "yes," "maybe").

One issue arose in the use of deictic terms like "here" in the phrase "over here" or "that" in the phrase "that one." Our final determination was to consider these deictic pronouns. One set of indefinite words was classified as pronouns as well ("something," "anything," "everything," etc.).

Note that items could well be double or even triple classified as the system permits numerous analyses that may involve the same item.

Lexical Problems

Because indefinite terms have been noted to contribute to empty speech (Nicholas et al., 1985) we counted indefinite words (e.g., "thing," "something," "anything"), many of which have been included as pronouns, as well.

Difficulties arose in determining neologisms that were intended to be single words as compared to extended jargon. Thus, "She was wearing /gEbz/ in" was considered a neologism, whereas "/džakiʌdẑaka/bringing one from the other" was considered jargon. Note that paragrammatic errors like "felled" were classified as paragrammatic but not as a neologisms in this system; a neologism had to have a nonword stem.

In our system, semantic and verbal paraphasias can only occur for content words. The only exception is that some pronouns when substituted (e.g., "she" for "he") were considered to be semantic paraphasias. Literal paraphasias, by contrast, could occur on both content and functor words. For example, a patient who said /də/ for "the" when the article "the" had been used correctly in other contexts was considered to have made a literal paraphasia in this instance. This was done to exclude dysarthric errors or dialectal variation from paraphasias.

SYNTAX

The interesting syntactic errors are the omissions characteristic of agrammatic patients and the substitution errors characteristic of paragrammatic patients. (For discussion of how these two are not necessarily as different as previously have been thought, see Heeschen, 1985, and Menn & Obler, 1990.) As Saffran et al. (1989) discussed, with respect to omissions, it is sometimes appealing to guess what a patient may have meant, but our rule, like theirs, is minimal reconstruction (as in Menn & Obler, 1990). For example, the phrase "this bad" with falling intonation on "bad" implying an entire sentence was intended, has clearly had an "is" omitted by a speaker of Standard English. If the subject says "cookie jar" with the same falling intonation, we know something has been omitted, but we cannot say what, so no codings are made for omissions in such an instance. Rather we code such an item as an instance of omission/fragment, but not more than one, even if probably more then one omitted word would have been intended. (For more examples of omissions, see Appendix C, p. 77.)

Paragrammatisms are considered in two forms: paragrammatisms involving whole words and paragrammatisms involving bound morphemes. Paragrammatisms involving whole words include misuse of functors, word order errors, and idiom errors (e.g., "Her mind is preoccupied"; "The sink is flowing the water"; "What's mining about her"; "There'll be a big bang hitting the boy from the cookie jar as the tripod is beginning to tilt and fall her"). In Appendix B, for example, our fluent subject says (lines 199–206), "One of them is trying to get it above the top." Because "top" cannot refer to the child's toy, and because it is hard (although not impossible!) to construe a situation in which this phrasing would be appropriate for a normal, we have labeled it *paragrammatic*.

Omissions were potentially of either substantives or functors that are obligatory, in line with the minimum reconstruction principle. See Appendix C, where our nonfluent subject, lines 8–14, says "Mother was dishes," for which two omissions are scored. No omission is scored for a possible "The" before *Mother*, as *Mother* may occur as a proper name without it in this situation. However, clearly some modification functors are missing for the verb (washes, or is washing), and an article may be missing before "dishes." Note that for this analysis omissions and fragments are labeled the same because we employ the Hier et al. (1985) definition "fragments are utterances complete in meaning but incomplete grammatically."

PRAGMATICS

One sort of pragmatic error relatively common in aphasic speech, is aposiopesis. For example, "I'm still, the mother is washing dishes" or "The dishes are, the boy is about to fall," "There's some collecting, he's about to let water . . ." or

(Appendix B, lines 149–162). Recall that what follows aposiopesis is unrelated to what preceded it, and that these sorts of false starts are different from those that terminate in the intended item.

The other sorts of pragmatic elements we set up coding for were included because they do occur in the narrative discourse of healthy elderly individuals, even on this limited task (Nicholas et al., 1985; Obler et al., chapter 2, this volume). The examples given in the appended handbook came either from our aphasics or from the normals.

It is our impression that curses or even exclamations such as "Jesus Christ" occur more often in aphasics then in normal subjects, at least in formal settings such as a hospital session with a clinician. What is interesting is that the other sorts of pragmatic behaviors (judgments, statements of unsureness, apology, personalization of the materials, and giving names to the characters in the picture) only occur among normal subjects. In one curious finding, giving names to the characters (e.g., "Johnny is reaching for the cookie jar") occurred in normals but not in patients with Alzheimer's dementia (Obler, Au, Litter, Freedman, & Albert, in preparation).

FINAL COMMENTS

Prior experience with prescriptive grammar in high school, and even in linguistics courses, had led us to expect that discourse parsing would be simple. Over and over, however, we have been struck with the difficulties in identifying category boundaries in terms of parts of speech, especially vis-à-vis functors, adverbs, adjectives, nonpersonal pronouns, and numbers. Difficult to classify words in idiomatic structures posed somewhat different problems because of our sense that idioms were being employed as units, rather than as strings of classifiable parts of speech. Assigning parts of speech for paragrammatic utterances also presented challenges, as functors were used inappropriately.

When coding utterances as paragrammatic, we found problems arose due to the vague definitions of pragrammatism in the literature, and due to a substantial number of instances in which the syntax felt "slightly off" but did not constitute a clear-cut error.

In addition, we experienced difficulty in some paragrammatic instances, in determining whether the error was due to a paraphasia for the substantive or a substitution for the functor. For example, in Appendix B, when this fluent patient says "The water is about to silk through" (lines 113–119), the word "silk" could be considered a verbal paraphasia, although it is unclear for what target, but likely "through" is a substitution as well, as we can think of no target for "silk" that would co-occur with "through."

Although we have extended systematic analysis beyond the frame Saffran et al. (1989) proposed for agrammatic utterances, we note that our analyses are appropriate for narrative discourse, but would be quite incomplete for analysis of conversational discourse. Although narrative discourse is used in daily life, and thus provides a functionally appropriate test of aphasic language production, we envision our approach to be one of many that should be used to study discourse in brain-damaged populations.

ACKNOWLEDGMENTS

This project was funded by NIH Grant #NS 25367-02. Our thanks also to Sandy Beckman for help in testing patients and Kelly Robinson for comments, suggestions, and word processing the handbook.

APPENDIX A: ORAL COOKIE THEFT ANALYSIS GUIDE[3]

The purpose of this analysis is to know how subjects build sentences and how complex those sentences are.

I. Transcription Notes

A. Listen to the tape and write as accurately as possible what you hear. Leave a 2" margin for examiner's utterances and any other comments.

B. Write in pencil because you need to listen to the narrative several times and edit. For possible neologisms and paraphasias, the rule of thumb is that any utterance which sounds like a real word should be transcribed as such.

C. This analysis is grammatical, not phonetic, so write out all morphological units. Write "going to," not "gonna."

D. Transcribe the entire narrative.

II. Analysis

Tips: It's a good idea to have the tape available while you're doing the analysis, so you can listen to any unintelligible or hard-to-categorize sections. The intonation contour of an utterance sometimes helps to categorize units, especially neologisms. Any unusual decisions on your part should be noted on the score sheet. Each item counted should be copied to the score sheet with its line number.

---

[3]This appendix is authored by Anita Haravon with Loraine K. Obler, prepared in consultation with Lisa Van Breedman, Janice Kugler, and Kelly Robinson.

A. MORPHOLOGY

1a. *Unit Total* (units include all repetitions, false starts, and fillers e.g. um, uh, well). Contractions are counted as two words. Write a running total of the unit count on the left side of the transcription). The number on the left side should refer to the number of the first unit on that line. This unit number will also be used for referencing subsequent items on the tally sheet, so it will be used as a "line reference number." Check your work at least once.

1b. *Units to First Prompt*

1c. *Narrative Time to First Prompt* (in seconds). Use a stopwatch to time the narrative from the end of the examiner's request, "Tell me the story of what's going on in this picture," to the beginning of the examiner's first prompt "Is there anything else you can/want/care to comment on?" Measure the narrative twice and take the average time to the nearest second.

1d. *Scoreability.* It will not be possible to linguistically analyze the monologues for some subjects. Their monologues will be classified as:

a. Unscoreable: Jargon + Stereotypies (automatic, empty speech)

b. Unscoreable: Jargon + Real Words (content words, meaningful)

c. Unscoreable: Real Word Repetition (irrelevant to task e.g.,"fish, fish, fish")

N.B. *Notation for Score Sheet.* The categories for analysis should be marked on the tally sheet in the following way:
example: Noun—clear-cut

1. mother	(7)
first noun in discourse	line reference number

Note: The following calculations are based on the narrative up to the first prompt only or the first 100 units (whichever comes first).

2. *Total Repetitions/False Starts/Repairs*
wavy dark blue line with arrow to final production
For the purposes of this analysis, repetitions, false starts, and repairs are all counted as one category. Write all occurences of false starts, each failed attempt should be counted because each attempt is a unit (e.g., "[ki] [ki] kitchen" is scored as two repetitions or failed attempts). Repetitions should be tallied under one category only (e.g., "get getting" is a word repetition, not a syllable repetition). Repetitions must be contiguous in the narrative (words that are uttered in a later sentence are not counted as repetitions). To calculate Total Repetitions, add Syllable, Word, and Phrase Repetitions (EXCLUDE Sentence Repetition).

2a. Syllable and Subsyllable Repetition ([s] [s] sitting)
wavy line *s* ("s" is subscripted)

2b. Word Repetition
wavy line *w*

i. word—literal (*in* .. in the cookie jar)

ii. word—nonliteral (I *could* .. *might* . . .)

2c. Phrase Repetition
wavy line *p*

i. phrase—literal (*in the* . . . in the cookie jar)

ii. phrase—nonliteral (*I could* .. I might)

2d. Sentence/Clause Repetition
no mark on transcription; not included in total

i. sentence—literal (do not have to be contiguous)

ii. sentence—nonliteral (counted only if inappropriate to discourse)

3. Total Fillers and Verbal Tics (uhm, well, like)
underline in green
4. Jargon (longer than neologism/extended units or global aphasia output)
wavy dark green line
5. Word Total
6. Stereotypies (words that are idiosyncratic to a particular subject) (e.g., "oh boy")
circle in pencil

The substantives and functors of all sentences should be tallied in the calculations below. For repetitions, count the final attempt only. If you aren't sure of the part of speech of a word, then look it up in the dictionary.
Note: Parts of Speech Clear-Cut vs. Questionable. The questionable category is used for words that can be classified as several parts of speech. For example (a) "He is doing *cooking* jar" "Cooking" is classified as verb questionable, adjective questionable, paragrammatism. (b) "She is trying to [kɔli] in the cookie jar." "[kɔli]" is classified as verb questionable, neologism. (c) "She is [wɔIr] water or something." "[wɔIr]" is classified as verb questionable, neologism. (d) "She seems to clean her arm." "Arm" is classified as semantic paraphasia questionable, verbal paraphasia questionable.

7. Substantives

7a. Nouns (including gerunds) (e.g., "washing dishes is boring")
underline dark blue

i. nouns—clearcut, e.g., 'boy'

ii. nouns—questionable

7b. Verbs (main verbs, infinitives, present participle, e.g., "He *falls* off"; "*washing* dishes")
underline red
i. verbs—clear-cut
ii. verbs—questionable

7c. Adjectives that are substantives (e.g., "cookie jar")
underline brown
i. adjectives—clear-cut
ii. adjectives—questionable

7d. Adverbs that are substantives (e.g., "slowly")
underline light green
i. adverbs—clear-cut
ii. adverbs—questionable

8. Total Functors

8a. Pronouns (e.g., "*He* is reaching for . . .")
circle in dark blue
i. pronouns—clear-cut
ii. pronouns—questionable

8b. Auxilary, Copula, and Modal Verbs (e.g., "*is* falling, is, want")
circle in dark orange

8c. Conjunctions
circle in black
i. and
ii. all other conjunctions (e.g., *as* when used to mean "because"; *so, therefore, however.* If a word can be scored as both a conjunction and an adverb, it should be scored as a conjunction)

8d. All Other Functors
circle in green
Includes all articles, prepositions, and words that just don't "feel" like substantives (e.g., yes, no, not, still, never)

9. Indefinite Words (e.g., thing, something, anything)
circle in light blue

Note: At this point every word should be tallied under some category. If a neologism, paraphasia, or paragrammatism occurs in a repeated segment it should be tallied under its respective category. For neologisms or paraphasias write what patient said and the target if known. If you are not certain of the utterance, it should be tallied under questionable neologism or questionable verbal paraphasia. Syllable repairs that seem to be neologisms or paraphasias can be ignored (e.g., "[rɔ] steal the old . . ."$_2$).

10. Neologism (nonword, not potentially related to target, *not* extended jargon)
    wavy light green line
    i. neologism—clear-cut (e.g. "[wIr]")
    ii. neologism—questionable
11. Paraphasias
    11a. Literal (nonword or real word, phonetically obviously related to target (e.g., [tUki] for "cookie")
        wavy dark orange line
        i. literal paraphasias—clear-cut
        ii. literal paraphasias—questionable
    11b. Semantic (real word, obviously semantically, but not phonetically related to target (e.g., "table" for "stool")
        wavy yellow line
        i. semantic paraphasias—clear-cut
        ii. semantic paraphasias—questionable
    11c. Verbal (real word, neither phonetically, nor semantically related to target (e.g., "send this one all over the *town* and she's standing in it")
        wavy red line
        i. verbal paraphasias—clear-cut
        ii. verbal paraphasias—questionable

B. SENTENCE LEVEL (the general rule is minimal reconstruction)
    1. Paragrammatism (misuse of functors, word order errors, idiom errors)
    1a. Unbound (e.g., "right *of* a wrong")
        red brackets
        i. unbound morpheme paragrammatism—clear-cut
        ii. unbound morpheme paragrammatism—questionable
    1b. Bound (e.g., "felled")
        red brackets
        i. bound morpheme paragrammatism—clear-cut
        ii. bound morpheme paragrammatism—questionable
    2. Omission (omission of substantives or functors, e.g., "instead of look{ing} so happy")
        green brackets
        i. omission—clearcut
        ii. omission—questionable
    3. Aposiopesis (abrupt termination of an utterance that leaves a thought incomplete from Hier et al., 1985, e.g., (a) "I am still, the mother is

washing the dishes" (b) "The dishes are, the boy is about to fall")
orange brackets

i. aposiopesis—clear-cut
ii. aposiopesis—questionable

C. SEMANTICS/THEMES (Could someone who has never seen the Cookie Theft Picture understand what was going on based on the subjects description?) Credit may be given for verbatim or synonymous mention of the items below. Partial credit may be given. Scoring: 1, .5, 0)

_____ Total # of themes subject referred to in description
circled in red
_____ # of first item subject referred to
_____ 1. mother/woman/lady
_____ 2. washing/wiping/drying/doing the dishes
_____ 3. water overflowing out of the sink
_____ 4. boy/kid
_____ 5. stealing/reaching for cookies
_____ 6. stool tipping/boy falling off the stool
_____ 7. girl/sister
_____ 8. mother not paying attention/oblivious
_____ 8a. First Connector: Mother doesn't notice children stealing cookies
red parentheses around whole sentence
_____ 8b. Second Connector: Mother doesn't notice sink overflowing
blue parentheses around whole sentence

D. PRAGMATICS

1. Judgments (e.g., "it looks particularly tranquil for such a mess going on")
light blue brackets
2. Unsureness (e.g., "I don't think . . . ," "I guess")
dark orange brackets
3. Apology (e.g., "I am sorry")
brown brackets
4. Egocentric Comment/Personalization (e.g., "He looks like my son")
purple brackets
5. Giving Names (e.g., "Johnny is reaching for the cookie")
light orange brackets
6. Other/Curses/Exclamations (e.g., "that's all I see," "damn," "Jesus Christ!")
grey brackets

III. Calculate totals and transfer to CODING SHEET for computer input.

APPENDIX B: MICROANALYSIS OF DISCOURSE IN APHASIC PATIENTS

A discourse sample from a fluent aphasic patient:

Examiner:
Tell me the story of what you see going on in this picture.

Patient:
1 Sure. (pause) well there's a a young
8 man a a boy baby a young
15 man, who is about to have a
22 have some cookies /ah/ and he's
29 trying to buy /ah/ get a wrist,
36 he's trying to get a piece, trying to,
45 trying to get the cookies but
51 he's about to fall over because
58 /ah/ he's unable to /ah/ he's going to
67 fall over and not, but he's
75 going to get two cookies
80 one of which is going to be
87 given to another little girl. Excuse me
94 /um/ while on the other end
100 the mother is /ah/ drilling some
106 /ah/ is pumping some water from it
113 but the water is about to
119 silk through, the water is
124 passing through the water and it's
131 going to make the whole place
137 sloppy and /wEDə/ wetter /um/ while,
143 let's see, the major types
149 of things here /ʌ/ there's some /ʌ/
157 collecting, he's about to
162 let the water /ra/ /pa/ /ʌ/, he's
170 about to lose, baby is, the
176 /saI/, the woman is about
181 to loose water from water
186 slopping through while the
190 children are on the side
195 getting some cookies. One
199 of them's trying to get it
206 above the top, from the top
212 and the other woman is
217 trying the other young
221 /wUm/ young girl
224 is trying to get some

	229	to help. That's about the best
	234	I can get out of this.
Anything else you want to comment on?	240	Very boring, very boring thing.

Time to first prompt: 100 sec.
Time to end: 103 sec.

NIH STUDY
ORAL COOKIE THEFT CODING SHEET

CODE B SUBJECT fluent TEST ____ Tallied by ah Date 12-31-91

A. Morphology

244 Unit Total 239 Units to First Prompt 100 Narrative Time

11 2. TOTAL REPETITIONS

0 Syllable Repetitions

5 Word Repetitions 2 literal 3 nonliteral

6 Phrase Repetitions 1 literal 5 nonliteral

0 Sentence Repetitions ____ literal ____ nonliteral

6 3. FILLER TOTAL 0 4. JARGON

discontinue 5. ~~WORD~~ TOTAL 0 6. STEREOTYPIES

18 7. TOTAL SUBSTANTIVES

6 NOUNS 6 definite 0 questionable

8 MAIN VERBS 8 definite 0 questionable

4 ADJECTIVES 4 definite 0 questionable

0 ADVERBS 0 definite 0 questionable

50 8. TOTAL FUNCTORS

13 PRONOUNS discontinue ~~Personal~~ ____ ~~Deictic~~ 13 definite 0 ques

[0 PRONOUNS without ANTECEDENT (do not add)]

12 AUXILIARY VERBS 12 definite 0 ques

5 CONJUNCTIONS TOTAL 2 and 3 all other conj. 0 ques

20 ALL OTHER FUNCTORS 20 definite 0 ques

Revised 6/18/90 AH

CODE 8 SUBJECT fluent TEST ____
Oral Cookie Theft CODING SHEET...page 2

0 9. INDEFINITE WORDS

0 10. NEOLOGISMS — 0 definite — 0 questionable

7 11. PARAPHASIAS

0 LITERAL	0 definite	0 questionable	
4 SEMANTIC	4 definite	0 questionable	
3 VERBAL	3 defintite	0 questionable	

B. SYNTAX

5 PARAGRAMMATISMS

4 UNBOUND	4 definite	0 questionable
1 BOUND	1 definite	0 questionable
0 OMISSIONS	0 definite	0 questionable
4 APOSIOPESIS	4 definite	0 questionable

C. SEMANTICS

5 TOTAL — 4 first story item

1 mother	0 washing dishes	.5 water overflowing	
1 boy	1 stealing cookies	.5 stool tipping	1 girl
0 mother oblivious	0 1st connector	0 2nd connector	

D. PRAGMATICS

0 Judgment	0 Unsureness	0 Apology
0 Personalization	0 Giving Names	1 Other

Oral Cookie Theft TALLY SHEET

CODE B

SUBJECT Fluent
TEST ____
Tallied by AH

Revised 6/18/90 AH

Date 12-13-91

A. Morphology
244 1a. Unit Total
239 1b. Units to First Prompt
100 1c. Narrative Time to First Prompt (in seconds)

Note: The following calculations are based on the narrative up to the first prompt, only. For each entry below, write the word and its line number from the transcription.

11 2. TOTAL Repetitions/False Starts (dark blue)
(not including sentence repetitions)

0 a. Syllable and Sub-syllable Repetition

5 b. Word Repetitions (wavy line w)
2 i. Word-Literal (in ..in the cookie jar)
1. a (1)
2. a (8)

3 ii. Word-NonLiteral (I could..might...)
① boy → baby (8) ② buy → get (29) ③ baby → a young man (8)

6 c. Phrase Repetitions (wavy line p)
1 i. Phrase-Literal (in the, in the cookie jar)
① trying to (36)

5 ii. Phrase-NonLiteral (I could..I might...)
① a young man → ② a boy → a young man (8) ③ have a → have some (15)
④ he's trying to get a wrist → ⑤ he's trying to get a piece → trying to get the cookies (45)

0 d. Sentence/Clause Repetitions (no marking on transcription)
0 i. Sentence-Literal

CODE B
SUBJECT Fluent

Oral Cookie Theft TALLY SHEET...page 2

0 ii. Sentence-NonLiteral

6 3. **Filler Total** (underline in green)

1. ah (22)
2. ah (29)
3. ah (58)
4. ah (58)
5. um (94)
6. well (1)

0 4. **Jargon** (wavy dark green line)

discontinue ~~5. **Word Total**: Count on transcription, excluding previously marked repetitions, fillers, and jargon.~~

0 6. **Stereotypies**

18 7. TOTAL **SUBSTANTIVES** (a-d) {N, Adj, Adv, Verb}

6 a. **Nouns** and Gerunds (dark blue)

6 i. Nouns-definite

1. man (15)
2. cookies (22)
3. cookies (45)
4. cookies (75)
5. girl (87)
6. end (94)

____ ii. Nouns-questionable

CODE B _ _
SUBJECT Fluent

Oral Cookie Theft TALLY SHEET...page 3

8 b. **Main Verbs**, Infinitives , and Present Participles (red)
8 i. Main Verbs-definite

1. have (22)
2. trying (45)
3. get (45)
4. fall (51)
5. fall (67)
6. get (75)
7. given (87)

0 ii. Main Verbs-questionable

4 c. **Adjectives that are Substantives** (brown)
4 i. Adjectives-definite (eg. cookie jar; is balanced)

1. young (8)
2. unable (58)
3. two (75)
4. little (87)

0 ii. Adjectives-questionable

0 d. **Adverbs that are Substantives** (light green)
0 i. Adverbs-definite (eg. slowly)

0 ii. Adverbs-questionable

50 8. Total # of FUNCTORS (a-d) {art, proN, aux, prep, conj, adj + adv}
13 a. TOTAL Pronouns and Deictic Terms (dark blue)
discontinue ~~i. Personal~~ ProN ~~ii.~~ Deictic ~~iii. Other~~

13 i. definite

1. there (1)
2. who (15)
3. some (22)
4. he (22)
5. he (51)
6. he (58)
7. he (58)
8. he (67)
9. one (80)
10. one (80)
11. another (87)
12. other (94)
13. me (87)

0 ii. questionable

CODE ___
SUBJECT Fluent

Oral Cookie Theft TALLY SHEET...page 4

__0__ iv. ProN w/o antecedent (dark blue with "?")
DO NOT ADD

__12__ b. Auxiliary, Copula, and Modal Verbs (dark orange)

__12__ i. questionable

1. is (15)
2. 's (22)
3. 's (51)
4. 's (58)
5. 's (58)
6. 's (67)
7. going (75)
8. is (80)
9. going (80)
10. be (80)
11. 's (1)
12. going (58)

__0__ ii. questionable

__5__ c. Conjunctions Total (black)

__2__ i. and

1. (22)
2. (67)

__3__ ii. all other conjunctions

1. but (45)
2. because (51)
3. but (67)

__0__ iii. questionable

__20__ d. All Other Functors (dark green)

__20__ i. definite

1. sure (1)
2. about (15)
3. to (15)
4. to (45)
5. the (45)
6. about (51)
7. to (51)
8. over (51)
9. to (58)
10. to (67)
11. over (67)
12. not (67)
13. to (75)
14. of (80)
15. to (80
16. to (87)
17. while (94)
18. on (94)
19. the (94)
20. the (100)

__0__ ii. questionable

CODE B
SUBJECT Fluent

Oral Cookie Theft TALLY SHEET...page 5

0 9. Indefinite Words (thing, something, anything) (circle light blue)

0 10. **Neologisms** (wavy light green line)
0 a. Neologisms-definite

0 b. Neologisms-questionable (add "?")

7 11. **Paraphasias**
0 a. **Literal** (wavy dark orange line)
0 i. Literal Paraphasias-definite

0 ii. Literal Paraphasias-questionable (add "?")

4 b. **Semantic** (wavy yellow line)
4 i. Semantic Paraphasias-definite (eg. "table" for "stool")

1. baby → boy (8)
2. buy → get (29)
3. piece → cookie (36)
4. he → she (157)

CODE B
SUBJECT Fluent

Oral Cookie Theft TALLY SHEET...page 6

0 ii. Semantic Paraphasias-questionable (add "?")

3 c. Verbal (wavy red line)
3 i. Verbal Paraphasias-defintite
1. wrist → piece (29) 3. silk (119) -> fall
2. dulling (100)

0 ii. Verbal Paraphasias-questionable (add"?")

B. SYNTAX [brackets]
5 1. Paragrammatism [red brackets] (functor, word order, idiom errors)
4 a. Unbound
4 i. Unbound Morpheme Paragrammatisms-definite
1. the water is passing through the water (119)
2. the water is about to silk through (113)
3. The woman is about to lose water from water slopping through (186)
4. One of them is trying to get above the top. (199)

0 ii. Unbound Morpheme Paragrammatisms-questionable (add "?")

1 b. Bound
1 i. Bound Morpheme Paragrammatisms-definite (eg. "felled")
1. The mother is pour [ ] some water from it. (106)

0 ii. Bound Morpheme Paragrammatisms-questionable (add "?")

0 2. Omission ([green brackets])
0 a. Omisssion-definite

CODE B
SUBJECT _

Oral Cookie Theft TALLY SHEET...page 7

__0__ b. Omission-questionable (add "?")

Aposiopesis

__4__ 3. ([orange brackets])

__4__ a. definite

1. He's about to fall over because he's unable to ___ (58)
2. He's going to fall over and not ___ (67)
3. There's some collecting of ___ (157)
4. He's about to let the water_ (162)

__0__ b. questionable

C. SEMANTICS (can give partial credit: 1.0, 0.5, 0.0)

__5__ TOTAL # of story items patient referred to (total=8: marked on transcript as circled number in red)

__4__ # of first story item referred to by patient

__1__ 1. mother/woman/lady
__0__ 2. washing/wiping/drying/doing dishes
__.5__ 3. water overflowing out of sink
__1__ 4. boy/kids
__1__ 5. stealing/reaching for cookies
__.5__ 6. stool tipping/ boy falling off stool
__1__ 7. girl/sister
__0__ 8. mother not paying attention/oblivious

linkage: __0__ 8a. First connector: Mother doesn't notice children (red)
__0__ 8b. Second connector: Mother doesn't notice sink overflowing (blue)

D. PRAGMATICS [brackets]

__0__ 1. Judgments (light blue brackets)

__0__ 2. Unsureness (dark orange brackets)

CODE B
SUBJECT fluent

Oral Cookie Theft TALLY SHEET...page 8

0 3. Apology (brown brackets)

0 4. Egocentric Comment-Personalization (purple brackets)

0 5. Giving Names (light orange brackets)

1 6. Other (grey brackets)
1. Excuse me.

E. COMMENTS

APPENDIX C: MICROANALYSIS OF DISCOURSE IN APHASIC PATIENTS

A discourse sample from a nonfluent aphasic patient:

Examiner:	Patient:	
Tell me the story of	1	uhm /g/ girl ah cookies ah mm
what you see going	8	uhm girl the cookies and mother
on in this picture.	14	ah /m/ wash dishes and uhm mhm
	21	oh mhm uhm
Anything else?	24	mother ah /w/ wash the the dishes
	31	and /d/ doesn't see and mh doesn't
	40	see oh the th- uhm uhm
	46	doesn't see water running ah ah under
	54	the floor and ah mh /m/ boy ah
	62	stand mhm mhm /m gm / /m gm /

Time to first prompt: 85 seconds
time to end: 183 seconds

NIH STUDY
ORAL COOKIE THEFT CODING SHEET

CODE C SUBJECT Nonfluent TEST ____ Tallied by KR Date 1/93

A. Morphology

66 Unit Total 23 Units to First Prompt 85 sec. Narrative Time

2 2. TOTAL REPETITIONS

2 Syllable Repetitions

0 Word Repetitions 0 literal 0 nonliteral

0 Phrase Repetitions 0 literal 0 nonliteral

0 Sentence Repetitions 0 literal 0 nonliteral

10 3. FILLER TOTAL 0 4. JARGON

discontinue 5. ~~WORD~~ TOTAL 0 6. STEREOTYPIES

7 7. TOTAL SUBSTANTIVES

6 NOUNS 6 definite 0 questionable

1 MAIN VERBS 1 definite 0 questionable

0 ADJECTIVES 0 definite 0 questionable

0 ADVERBS 0 definite 0 questionable

3 8. TOTAL FUNCTORS

0 PRONOUNS discontinue ~~Per~~sonal ____ ~~Deict~~ic 0 definite 0 questionable

[0 PRONOUNS without ANTECEDENT (do not add)]

0 AUXILIARY VERBS 0 definite 0 questionable

2 CONJUNCTIONS TOTAL 2 and 0 all other conj. 0 ques

1 ALL OTHER FUNCTORS 1 definite 0 questionable

Revised 6/18/90 AH

CODE <u>C</u> SUBJECT <u>Non fluent</u> TEST ____
Oral Cookie Theft <u>CODING</u> SHEET...page 2

<u>0</u> 9. INDEFINITE WORDS <u>0</u> def <u>0</u> ques

<u>0</u> 10. NEOLOGISMS <u>0</u> definite <u>0</u> questionable

<u>0</u> 11. PARAPHASIAS

<u>0</u> LITERAL <u>0</u> definite <u>0</u> questionable

<u>0</u> SEMANTIC <u>0</u> definite <u>0</u> questionable

<u>0</u> VERBAL <u>0</u> defintite <u>0</u> questionable

B. SYNTAX

<u>0</u> PARAGRAMMATISMS

<u>0</u> UNBOUND <u>0</u> definite <u>0</u> questionable

<u>0</u> BOUND <u>0</u> definite <u>0</u> questionable

<u>2</u> OMISSIONS <u>2</u> definite <u>0</u> questionable

<u>0</u> APOSIOPESIS <u>0</u> definite <u>0</u> questionable

C. SEMANTICS

<u>3</u> TOTAL <u>7</u> first story item

<u>1</u> mother <u>1</u> washing dishes <u>0</u> water overflowing

<u>0</u> boy <u>0</u> stealing cookies <u>0</u> stool tipping <u>1</u> girl

<u>0</u> mother oblivious <u>0</u> 1st connector <u>0</u> 2nd connector

D. PRAGMATICS

<u>0</u> Judgment <u>0</u> Unsureness <u>0</u> Apology

<u>0</u> Personalization <u>0</u> Giving Names <u>0</u> Other

Oral Cookie Theft TALLY SHEET

CODE C

SUBJECT NonFluent
TEST ____
Tallied by KR

Revised 6/18/90 AH

Date 1/93

A. Morphology

66 1a. Unit Total
23 1b. Units to First Prompt
85 1c. Narrative Time to First Prompt (in seconds)

Note: The following calculations are based on the narrative up to the first prompt, only. For each entry below, write the word and its line number from the transcription.

2 2. TOTAL Repetitions/False Starts (dark blue)
(not including sentence repetitions)

2 a. Syllable and Sub-syllable Repetition
1. g-girl (1) 2. m - wash (14)

0 b. Word Repetitions (wavy line w)
0 i. Word-Literal (in ..in the cookie jar)

0 ii. Word-NonLiteral (I could..might...)

0 c. Phrase Repetitions (wavy line p)
0 i. Phrase-Literal (in the, in the cookie jar)

0 ii. Phrase-NonLiteral (I could..I might...)

0 d. Sentence/Clause Repetitions (no marking on transcription)
0 i. Sentence-Literal

CODE C
SUBJECT NonFluent

Oral Cookie Theft TALLY SHEET...page 2

0 ii. Sentence-NonLiteral

10 3. **Filler** **Total** (underline in green)

1. uhm (1) 4. uhm (8) 7. uhm (14) 10. uhm (21)
2. ah (1) 5. ah (14) 8. oh (21)
3. ah (1) 6. uhm (14) 9. mhm (21)

0 4. **Jargon** (wavy dark green line)

discontinue 5. ~~**Word**~~ **Total**: Count on transcription, excluding previously marked repetitions, fillers, and jargon.

0 6. **Stereotypies**

7 7. TOTAL **SUBSTANTIVES** (a-d) {N, Adj, Adv, Verb}

6 a. **Nouns** and Gerunds (dark blue)

6 i. Nouns-definite

1. girl (1) 4. cookies (8)
2. cookies (1) 5. mother (8)
3. girl (8) 6. dishes (14)

0 ii. Nouns-questionable

CODE C
SUBJECT Nonfluent

Oral Cookie Theft TALLY SHEET...page 3

1 b. **Main Verbs**, Infinitives , and Present Participles (red)
1 i. Main Verbs-definite

1. wash (14)

0 ii. Main Verbs-questionable

0 c. **Adjectives that are Substantives** (brown)
0 i. Adjectives-definite (eg. cookie jar; is balanced)

0 ii. Adjectives-questionable

0 d. **Adverbs that are Substantives** (light green)
0 i. Adverbs-definite (eg. slowly)

0 ii. Adverbs-questionable

0 8. Total # of FUNCTORS (a-d) {art, proN, aux, prep, conj, adj + adv}
0 a. TOTAL Pronouns and Deictic Terms (dark blue)
~~i. Personal ProN~~ ~~ii. Deictic~~ ~~iii. Other~~
0 i. definite
0 ii. questionable

CODE C
SUBJECT NonFluent

Oral Cookie Theft TALLY SHEET...page 4

0 iv. ProN w/o antecedent (dark blue with "?")
DO NOT ADD

0 b. Auxiliary, Copula, and Modal Verbs (dark orange)
0 i. definite 0 ii. questionable

2 c. Conjunctions Total (black)
2 i. and
1. and (8)
2. and (14)

0 ii. all other conjunctions

0 iii. questionable

1 d. All Other Functors (dark green)
1 i. definite 0 ii. questionable
1. the (8)

CODE C
SUBJECT [illegible]

Oral Cookie Theft TALLY SHEET...page 5

0 9. Indefinite Words (thing, something, anything) (circle light blue) 0 def 0 ques

0 10. **Neologisms** (wavy light green line)
0 a. Neologisms-definite

0 b. Neologisms-questionable (add "?")

0 11. **Paraphasias**
0 a. **Literal** (wavy dark orange line)
0 i. Literal Paraphasias-definite

0 ii. Literal Paraphasias-questionable (add "?")

0 b. **Semantic** (wavy yellow line)
0 i. Semantic Paraphasias-definite (eg. "table" for "stool")

0 ii. Semantic Paraphasias-questionable (add "?")

0 c. **Verbal** (wavy red line)
0 i. Verbal Paraphasias-defintite

0 ii. Verbal Paraphasias-questionable (add"?")

B. SYNTAX [brackets]
0 1. **Paragrammatism** [red brackets] (functor, word order, idiom errors)
0 a. **Unbound**
0 i. Unbound Morpheme Paragrammatisms-definite

0 ii. Unbound Morpheme Paragrammatisms-questionable (add "?")

0 b. **Bound**
0 i. Bound Morpheme Paragrammatisms-definite (eg. "fell<u>ed</u>")

0 ii. Bound Morpheme Paragrammatisms-questionable (add "?")

2 2. **Omission** ([green brackets])
2 a. Omisssion-definite
1. mother [ ] wash (8-14)
2. wash [ ] dishes (14)

CODE C
SUBJECT NonFluent

Oral Cookie Theft TALLY SHEET...page 7

__0__ b. Omission-questionable (add "?")

__0__ 3. Aposiopesis ([orange brackets])
__0__ a. -definite

__0__ b. -questionable

C. SEMANTICS (can give partial credit: 1.0, 0.5, 0.0)

__3__ TOTAL # of story items patient referred to (total=8: marked on transcript as circled number in red)

__7__ # of first story item referred to by patient
__1__ 1. mother/woman/lady
__1__ 2. washing/wiping/drying/doing dishes
__0__ 3. water overflowing out of sink
__0__ 4. boy/kids
__0__ 5. stealing/reaching for cookies
__0__ 6. stool tipping/ boy falling off stool
__1__ 7. girl/sister
__0__ 8. mother not paying attention/oblivious

linkage: __0__ 8a. First connector: Mother doesn't notice children (red)
__0__ 8b. Second connector: Mother doesn't notice sink overflowing (blue)

D. PRAGMATICS [brackets]
__0__ 1. Judgments (light blue brackets)

__0__ 2. Unsureness (dark orange brackets)

CODE C
SUBJECT NonFluent

Oral Cookie Theft TALLY SHEET...page 8

0 3. Apology (brown brackets)

0 4. Egocentric Comment-Personalization (purple brackets)

0 5. Giving Names (light orange brackets)

0 6. Other (grey brackets)

E. COMMENTS

APPENDIX D: COOKIE THEFT PICTURE
from Boston Diagnostic Aphasia Examination
Goodglass & Kaplan, 1972

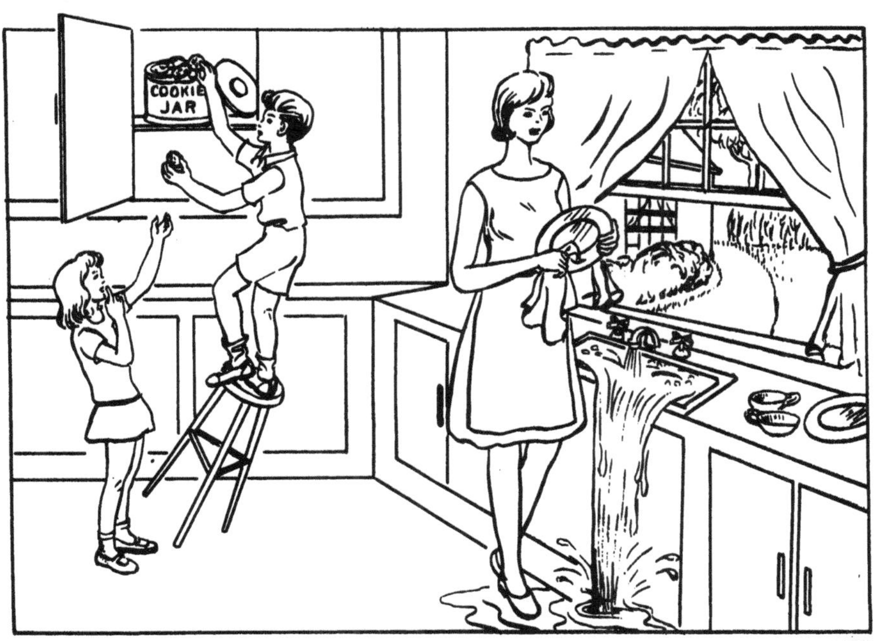

REFERENCES

Bloom, R. L. (1990). *Dissolution of discourse in patients with unilateral brain damage*. Unpublished doctoral dissertation, City University of New York.

Ehrlich, J. S. (1990). *Influence of structure on the content of oral narrative in adults with dementia of the Alzheimer's type*. Unpublished doctoral dissertation, City University of New York.

Ehrlich, J. S., Obler, L. K., Clark, L., Gerstman, L. J. (1993). *Influence of structure on narrative production in adults with dementia of the Alzheimer's type*. Manuscript submitted for review.

Goodglass, H., & Kaplan, E. (1972). *The assessment of aphasia and related disorders*. Philadelphia: Lea & Febiger.

Heeschen, C. (1985). Agrammatism versus paragrammatism: A fictitious opposition. In M. L. Kean (Ed.), *Agrammatism* (pp. 207–248). New York: Academic Press.

Hier, D. B., Hagenlocker, K., & Shindler, A. G. (1985). Language disintegration in dementia: Effects of etiology and severity. *Brain and Language, 25*, 117–133.

Menn, L., & Obler, L. K. (1990). *Agrammatic aphasia: A cross-language narrative sourcebook*. Amsterdam: Benjamins.

Nicholas, M., Obler, L. K., Albert, M. L., & Helm-Estabrooks, N. (1985). Empty speech in Alzheimer's disease and fluent aphasia. *Journal of Speech & Hearing Research, 28*, 405–410.

Obler, L. K., Au, R., Litter, J., Freedman, M., & Albert, M. L. (in preparation). *Agraphic errors in aging and dementia*.

Saffran, E. M., Berndt, R. S., & Schwartz, M. F. (1989). The quantitative analysis of agrammatic production: Procedure and data. *Brain and Language, 37*, 440–479.

Utlatowska, H., Freedman-Sterm, R., Doyel, A., Macaluso-Haynes, S., & North, S. (1983). Production of narrative discourse in aphasia. *Brain and Language, 13*, 345–371.

Chapter 5

Hemispheric Responsibility and Discourse Production: Contrasting Patients With Unilateral Left and Right Hemisphere Damage

Ronald L. Bloom
Hofstra University

In the classical explanation of the central language mechanism, the left cerebral hemisphere contains the neural structures that are responsible for processing words and sentences. To this day, the left-hemisphere explanation proposed by Karl Wernicke in 1874 remains the most accepted model of the central language-processing mechanism (Buckingham, 1982). However, converging neurobehavioral evidence has precipitated modification of the classical model by demonstrating that neuroanatomic structures in the left-hemisphere area do not function in isolation from other parts of the brain.

Word and sentence processing, the bases of the classical model, do not fully account for the contextual aspects of language. By contrast, examination of discourse production provides an abundant source of data for investigating the cognitive and social factors that enter into language. Discourse production includes word selection, sentence formation, organization of information, linking sentences with ideas, and deciding what should be said and what should remain unsaid. Examination of discourse provides an optimal opportunity for describing language as a dynamic and complex behavior that may be affected by the context in which it occurs.

This chapter reviews research that has examined discourse in patients with either unilateral left- or right-brain damage in order to clarify theories about hemispheric responsibility and the production of discourse. Insult to the brain disrupts the orderly interactions of the cognitive, social, and linguistic systems that contribute to normal discourse production. Following unilateral left- or right-brain damage the capacities of the two hemispheres become differentiated.

Analysis of discourse production in these two clinical populations provides a window for understanding the overlapping and interconnected neural networks distributed throughout the brain. After describing and comparing what is known about discourse in left-brain-damaged and right-brain-damaged subjects, a preliminary model of discourse production is proposed. The model represents an effort to account for the hemispheric-dependent mechanisms used in language production and their complementary responsibilities in discourse. Following the rationale for the development of this model, the clinical implications of the reported findings and the model derived from them are discussed.

DISCOURSE AND LEFT-BRAIN DAMAGE

A variety of elicitation techniques and evaluation procedures have been used to explore the discourse produced by different clinical groups of aphasic left-brain-damaged patients. A story-recall task enabled Berko Gleason and colleagues (1980) to describe differences in the narrative style among Broca's patients, Wernicke's patients, and normal controls. Overall, aphasic left-brain-damaged patients demonstrated a reduction in the number of meaningful themes recalled in their discourse and an absence of anaphora. Narratives of Broca's subjects contained fewer words and a preference for nouns over verbs. Wernicke's subjects were distinguished by the use of many words, an abundance of deictic terms, more verbs than nouns, and many concatenated sentences in place of embedded sentences. Berko Gleason and colleagues noted that aphasic subjects typically paraphrase a major theme several times and tend to neglect less salient parts of the story.

Procedures to quantify the discourse changes of recovering aphasic patients were developed by Yorkston and Beukelman (1980). Verbal picture descriptions from mild to moderate aphasic speakers were compared to those of normal adults on the basis of amount of information (content units) and efficiency (syllables per minute and content units per minute). Although there was an inverse relationship between aphasia severity and the amount of information produced, mild and moderate aphasics tended to express as much information as the normal speakers. According to Yorkston and Beukelman, it is the efficiency of the communication, not the amount of information conveyed, that distinguishes mild and moderate aphasic subjects from normal controls.

Ulatowska, North, and Macaluso-Haynes (1981) described the abilities of mildly impaired aphasics and age-matched normal speakers to produce procedural and narrative discourse. The recalled narratives of aphasic subjects were reported to be shorter and simpler than those of the nonaphasic subjects. Aphasics maintained the essential elements of story structure, preserved the chronological order of events, and omitted elements that did not affect plot development. Ulatowska and colleagues proposed that the discourse errors of mildly impaired aphasic subjects were also found to a lesser degree in the discourse of normals.

In a later study, Ulatowska, Freedman-Stern, Doyel, Macaluso-Haynes, and North (1983) described the abilities of moderately impaired aphasics and age-matched normals to retell a narrative, summarize it, and interpret the moral of the story. Consistent with their earlier findings for mildly impaired aphasics (Ulatowska et al., 1981), results showed that moderately impaired aphasics maintained the essential elements of narrative structure. In comparison to the normal controls, narratives of the moderately impaired aphasics were reduced in both quantity and complexity of language with errors most apparent at the sentence level. When the anterior and posterior aphasic patients in this study were compared, the posterior patients tended to produce more language, but no other differences in performance were revealed.

Narrative structure of aphasic patients was also investigated by Ernest-Baron, Brookshire, and Nicholas (1987), who had subjects listen to and retell two narrative stories three times in succession. Both aphasic and nonaphasic subjects retold a greater proportion of information units that were central to the story structure than information units that were peripheral to the story structure. Amount of information recalled across the three trials was noted to increase in both groups. Nonaphasic subjects always retold more information than aphasic subjects, although the differences were never statistically significant. Both subject groups preserved the order of information recalled across the three trials. Ernest-Baron et al. (1987) also noted that groups representing anterior and posterior syndromes of aphasia performed similarly on the experimental tasks.

A picture story task was used by Bloom, Borod, and Obler (1993) to examine the linguistic devices employed by mildly impaired left-brain-damaged aphasic patients to generate discourse. In comparison to normal controls, aphasic patients produced a limited range of connective forms, and demonstrated a reliance on the conjunction "and," the semantically least marked connective. The absence of other more complex connective forms (e.g., "but," "then") suggests limitations in the unity and temporal relatedness of the sentences in their discourse. In general, the left-brain-damaged patients interjected many extraneous remarks and tended to repeat words and phrases. The left-brain-damaged patients also produced more pronouns without antecedents and used many more deictic terms than the normal controls. Excessive use of these linguistic devices would render discourse vague and ambiguous. Bloom et al. (1993) noted that patients with both anterior and posterior left-hemisphere damage did not use connectives or anaphora appropriately in their discourse.

In summary, studies that have evaluated discourse production of mildly and moderately impaired left-brain-damaged aphasic subjects reveal a preservation of the global aspects of discourse structure. The similarity between aphasic and nonaphasic subjects in maintaining the global organization of discourse is surprising in face of the group differences in the use of phonology, syntax, and semantics. Although aphasic individuals produce narratives without compromising the essential elements of discourse, their narratives are less complex and lack certain cohesive devices. For example, Berko Gleason et al. (1980) and Bloom et al. (1993) noted that in comparison to normal subjects, aphasics often produced pronouns without identifying the referent. Ulatowska et al. (1981) noted aphasics use a higher percentage of definite articles for the first mention of nouns and characters in the narratives than do normal subjects. This may demonstrate insensitivity on the part of aphasic speakers to the rules that express understanding of a listener's perspective or reference. In addition, aphasic subjects have been found to shift verb tenses more frequently than normals and produce a restricted range of conjunctions (Berko Gleason et al., 1980; Bloom et al., 1993; Ulatowska et al., 1981). Inappropriate use of these cohesive devices signifies a disruption in the aphasic's knowledge of the way linguistic elements in a discourse are linked together. A noteworthy result of these discourse studies is the similarity reported between aphasic and normal control subjects and among groups with different syndromes of aphasia. Future research examining discourse production in aphasia will need to include a larger number of patients so that intrahemispheric location may be examined more closely and lesion size considered. Interhemispheric contrasts also reveal some remarkable differences in discourse production.

DISCOURSE AND RIGHT-BRAIN DAMAGE

Even in individuals who are left-hemisphere dominant for language, injury to the right side of the brain can cause selected deficits in discourse production. Research on the discourse of right-brain-damaged patients has resulted in several hypotheses proposed to explain the factors that mediate these deficits. Rivers and Love (1980), for example, asserted that disturbed visuospatial processing underlies the language performance of patients with right-brain damage. To test this hypothesis, they administered a set of visuospatial processing tests such as fragmented picture naming and storytelling from pictorial stimuli to right-brain-damaged subjects, left-brain-damaged subjects, and normal controls. Trained raters were employed to judge the fluency, articulation, semantics, and syntax of the subjects during the storytelling task. The raters consistently judged the right-brain-damaged subjects as having communication difficulties that exceeded those of the aphasic subjects. Because the patients with right-brain damage also performed poorly on the visuospatial processing tasks, Rivers and Love concluded that language following right-brain damage reflects deficits associated with the right hemisphere's contribution to visual perceptual processing.

Impairment in the appreciation and production of emotional information has also been hypothesized to account for the right-brain-damaged patients' discourse problems. Gardner, Brownell, Wapner, and Michelow (1983) examined right-brain-damaged patients on tasks of complex linguistic processing. These tasks were designed to assess subjects' abilities to recall narratives that were composed of spatial, emotional, and bizarre elements. Each subject listened to three versions of the same narrative that were elaborated through the insertion of either spatial, emotional, or bizarre story elements. After hearing each version of the story, subjects were asked to retell it in as much detail as possible. Results showed that the story recall of the right-brain-damaged subjects differed from that of the normal subjects in that emotional elements tended to trigger inappropriate embellishments. The right-brain-damaged subjects also demonstrated difficulty in reacting appropriately to the bizarre story elements.

Abilities in narrative organization in right-brain-damaged subjects have been investigated by Huber and Gleber (1982). In their study, left- and right-brain-damaged patients were required to arrange a set of picture cards and a set of written sentences into a story. The right-brain-damaged patients showed more difficulty arranging pictures than sentences. By contrast, left-brain-damaged aphasic patients demonstrated more difficulty arranging the written sentences. Because of the apparent dichotomy between visuospatial and linguistic processing skills in these groups of patients, the authors suggest that right-brain-damaged subjects and left-brain-damaged subjects rely on different strategies to organize narratives.

Delis, Wapner, Gardner, and Moses (1983) also investigated the narrative abilities of right-brain-damaged subjects and found results similar to those of Huber and Gleber (1982). Delis et al. demonstrated that right-brain-damaged patients had greater difficulty than did normal controls in performing a task requiring subjects to organize scrambled sentences into a story. That right-brain-damaged subjects present deficits in integrating sentences into a coherent narrative suggested that these subjects fail to utilize the surrounding linguistic context as they produce discourse.

Using a pictorial sequence of a story to elicit discourse, Joanette, Goulet, Ska, and Nespoulous (1986) evaluated the amount of information in the oral narratives of right-brain-damaged subjects and normal controls. Overall, the right-brain-damaged subjects' narratives contained less content and appeared to be a reduction of the information in the normal control's narratives. However, Joanette et al. noted that it is not clear whether the narrative deficits that result from right-brain damage represent a linguistic or cognitive problem or reflect visual perceptual deficits.

In order to examine the factors that mediate the discourse problems of right-brain-damaged subjects, Bloom, Borod, Obler, and Gerstman (1992) developed a picture story test to elicit discourse that contained either emotional, visuospatial, or neutral content. Right-brain-damaged, left-brain-damaged, and normal control right-handed adults were tested. Discourse analysis demonstrated that the number of words produced was equivalent for each subject group. However, both the right-brain-damaged and left-brain-damaged subjects expressed quantitatively less content than did the normal controls. When condition-related differences were examined within each group, there were no differences between left-brain-damaged subjects and normal controls. By contrast, the right-brain-damaged subjects showed a selective deficit when producing stories with emotional content. Because Bloom et al. controlled for visual perceptual, temporal, and cognitive deficits among subjects, findings suggested that the right hemisphere plays a special role in the production of discourse, especially when the content is emotional. Bloom et al. concluded that the right hemisphere, along with the left, is involved in producing the conceptual aspects of discourse.

In a second study, Bloom, Borod, Obler, and Gerstman (1993) used the picture story test to examine the effect of emotional content on the verbal pragmatic aspects of discourse production in right-brain-damaged, left-brain-damaged, and normal control adults. Stories were rated by three trained judges in order to determine appropriate use of seven verbal pragmatic features (e.g., conciseness, relevancy) of discourse. Across all three story conditions (emotional, visuospatial, and neutral), the brain-damaged groups were judged to be impaired relative to the normal controls. In the visuospatial and neutral conditions, left-brain-damaged subjects were found to be particularly pragmatically impaired, whereas in the emotional condition, right-brain-damaged subjects demonstrated significant pragmatic deficits. This analysis suggested that the pragmatic component of the language system interacts with the type of content expressed in discourse. Specifically, emotional content appeared to facilitate pragmatic performance among left-brain-damaged subjects and to suppress pragmatic performance among right-brain-damaged subjects. Results suggest that right-brain-damaged patients' problems with discourse production lie in their inability to maintain pragmatic organization at the suprasentential level.

In a third study in this series, Bloom, Borod, and Obler (1993) examined certain measures of discourse structure in order to understand the formal rules or linguistic devices employed by left- and right-brain-damaged patients to organize discourse. When compared to normal controls, the right-brain-damaged subjects produced errors that disrupted the cohesiveness of discourse organization. For example, right-brain-damaged subjects, rather than normal controls, produced more referential terms that did not have a clear referent. Specifically, right-brain-damaged patients used more pronouns without antecedents, more indefinite terms, more deictic terms, and more definite articles. Ambiguous use of these referential terms suggests a disruption in the perspective that a speaker shares with the listener. This finding is consistent with reports in the clinical literature (Gardner, 1975; Perecman, 1983) that suggest the speech of right-brain-damaged patients is often vague and nonspecific.

SUMMARY

The language deficits resulting from left-brain damage and right-brain damage are clearly two distinct clincial syndromes. Whereas the linguistic structure of the left-brain-damaged subjects generally becomes fragmented at the word and sentence level, the breakdown in right-brain-damaged subjects' discourse lies in processing larger language units that are informational or related to the organizing scheme that conveys the meaning of utterances to the listener.

Review of the literature strongly suggests that the discourse of the left-brain-damaged patients reflects the cognitive style of the unimpaired right hemisphere. For example, left-brain-damaged patients are able to take advantage of emotional content, emphasize their messages, and generate an internal representation of story structure. Similarly, the discourse of the right-brain-damaged patients seems to reflect the linguistic capacities of the unimpaired left hemisphere but is impoverished in the particular cognitive style of the right hemisphere. Specifically, the right-brain-damaged subjects are able to produce the sequential aspects of linguistic form but are impaired in simultaneously producing certain aspects of discourse structure. Unaware of their deficits, the right-brain-damaged subjects demonstrate a dependency on immediate context and a dissolution of the rules that permit speakers to share perspective with their communication partner. Results clearly suggest that in addition to specialized left-hemispheric linguistic abilities, discourse production involves cognitive processes that require both hemispheres of the brain.

TOWARD A MODEL OF DISCOURSE PRODUCTION

Contemporary models of language production have moved beyond descriptions of clinical syndromes in an effort to develop theories that account for both normal and pathological linguistic behaviors. Numerous models of language processing in normal and disordered speakers have been developed to account for single word reading (e.g., Morton, 1985), sentence production (e.g., Garrett, 1980), and agrammatism (e.g., Saffran, 1982). Typically, these models are composed of discrete components of the semantic or syntactic system organized into hierarchical levels. Construction of these models is based on observable dissociations between spared and impaired components of a speaker's language.

Whereas word and sentence-level descriptions are appropriately treated by componential models of linguistic processing, descriptions of discourse production must account for the capacities of the larger language system. The research just reviewed demonstrated that discourse production requires complementary hemispheric activity that can best be described as a series of synergistic processes. Thus, a model of discourse production should not only focus on identifying the components of discourse but also on how these components interact with each other. The model developed here has been titled the Synergistic Model of Discourse Production because it focuses on the simultaneous action of separate but cooperative components.

Clearly, a model of discourse production must take into account both left- and right-hemispheric processes. Several factors need to be considered in such a model. One critical factor is that both the left and right hemisphere are required to produce discourse that is fully informative (Bloom et al., 1992). Although the sentential aspects of language are preserved, the narratives of patients with right-brain damage are reduced in information especially when the content of the stories is emotional (Bloom et al., 1992). Left-brain-damaged patients also demonstrated a reduction in the amount of information used to tell stories but quantity of information was not influenced by the type of content expressed (Bloom et al., 1992). When the formal aspects of discourse production (i.e., use of specific linguistic devices that govern the organization of discourse) are considered, left-brain-damaged patients and right-brain-damaged patients both demonstrate a breakdown in the rules that establish reference between a speaker and a listener and a reduction in the use of strategies that may be employed to link sentences together (Bloom, Borod, & Obler, 1993). This observation is consistent with the view that both hemispheres make contributions to intersentential discourse organization. Interestingly, in both groups of brain-damaged patients, the type of content produced had no significant impact on the intersentential forms used to organize discourse. By contrast, the verbal pragmatic rules used by patients with left-brain damage and right-brain damage were significantly affected by the type of content expressed. The double dissociation observed when emotional content was examined is another factor that should be considered. Specifically, emotional content facilitated pragmatic performance among left-brain-damaged patients but suppressed these aspects of pragmatic performance among right-brain-damaged patients (Bloom, Borod, Obler, & Gerstman, 1993).

To account for the factors previously summarized, the model of discourse production proposed here (see Fig. 5.1) describes simultaneous and successive processing networks and the interaction of these components that delimit linguistic form (phonology, low-level semantics, syntax), content (high-level semantics), and the verbal aspects of pragmatics. The components of discourse are posited on the basis that they are autonomous and exist independently of each other. Components and networks that comprise the model have been labeled with initials and are cross referenced in Fig. 5.1 and in the text.

Components have been assigned to the simultaneous processing network (SPs) if a lesion in either hemisphere disrupts the function of that particular component. Components have been assigned to the successive processing network (SCs) if a disruption in that component arises solely from a unilateral left hemisphere lesion. This model of discourse production acknowledges that basic linguistic functions (i.e., phonology, morphology, syntax, and low-level semantics) are mediated primarily by the left hemisphere. The right hemisphere, by contrast, is a simultaneous processor. Discourse production is viewed as a unitary cognitive process, with right-hemisphere cognitive processing being supported by simultaneous and successive left-hemisphere processes. This accounts for the coexistence of widely distributed neural regions for the production of language in context and a highly specialized left-hemisphere language zone.

In this preliminary model, a unit of discourse is generated on the basis of input to any one of the simultaneous processors (SPs). The pragmatic component (PM) implements the verbal pragmatic rules that describe what a speaker needs

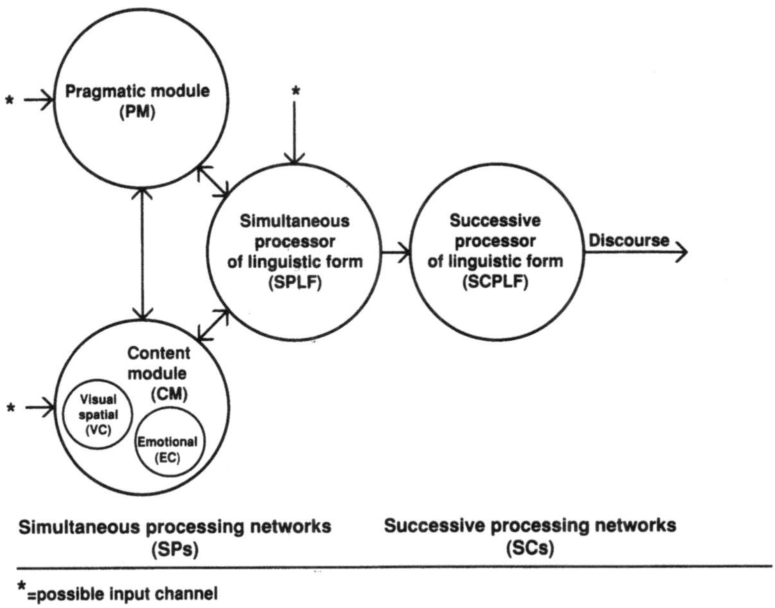

FIG. 5.1. Synergistic model of discourse production.

to do in order to convey a message to the listener. A request for a story may activate the pragmatic module where speakers construct information on the basis of what they think the listener needs to know. When the information is visuospatial or emotional, the content module (CM) may serve as the source of input. The simultaneous processor of linguistic form (SPLF) may serve as the input source when speakers have heard the story before or when they exploit prior knowledge of story structure (e.g., procedural discourse). Regardless of the source of input, the verbal pragmatic rules are processed simultaneously with other general cognitive functions and are defined over the entire unit of discourse.

A minimum of two content components that process specific cognitive structure are posited. So far only visuospatial content (VC) and emotional content (EC) components have been delimited. Visuospatial and emotional content have been delimited because deficits in these areas may occur independently of linguistic deficits (Walsh, 1987). Both of these components regulate specific aspects of higher level semantic processing and closely interact with the Pragmatic Module. Both content components (VC, EC) also reflect general cognitive function (e.g., processing emotional information) and may trigger compensatory adjustments within the pragmatic language system.

The formal rules of discourse structure are best understood as a pair of coexisting modules that differ in the type of processing they do and the way they interact with other modules. Together these modules represent the rules that regulate the possible structure of language. One of these formal modules is an

SPLF that connects linguistic form to the pragmatic module (PM). This module generates the rules that account for a speaker's representation of story structure. The second formal module (SCPLF) successively processes linguistic form (i.e., phonology, low-level semantics, syntax) and interconnects with the first formal module (SPLF). The connection between the two formal modules (SPLF and SCPLF) accounts for a speaker's ability to relate form and context, while maintaining the autonomy of the phonological and syntactic processing system. However, only the SPLF module is connected to the content module (CM). To account for the observed dissociation in linguistic form and high-level semantic content in brain-damaged patients (Bloom, Borod, & Obler, 1993), there is no direct interaction between the CM and the module that successively processes linguistic form (SCPLF).

For all adults, incoming stimuli (e.g., a request for a story) are evaluated through any of the simultaneous processors (CM, PM, SPLF). Based on either a speaker's experience in social contexts, the nature of the request or the speaker's notion of story structure, the verbal rules that convey intention are constructed and activated continuously over the discourse unit.

Following injury to the left hemisphere there is often a disruption in the second formal module (SCPLF). Output is thus characterized by successive processing deficits that manifest themselves as impairments in utilizing particular aspects of linguistic form (e.g., some anterior aphasia syndromes). This disruption may also impede the function of the first formal module resulting in impairments in generating a story structure and in using words to establish reference within a text (e.g., some posterior aphasia syndromes). Following left-brain damage, emotional cognitive structure (EC), stored in one of the CMs, is spared and through general cognitive processing, pragmatic competence may be activated. Overall, damage to the left hemisphere appears to mask pragmatic competence. Although there is evidence of preserved intention in the discourse of the left-brain-damaged patients, they are without the linguistic means necessary to accomplish their communicative goal. The reduction of content in the left-brain-damaged patients' discourse appears to be selective or self-regulated. Without the ability to execute the form of language successively, their discourse becomes laden with repetitions and attempts to complete their pragmatic goal are often futile.

Following right-brain damage, the cognitive structure of the CMs (i.e., visuospatial and emotional information) is often disrupted. Research reviewed here suggests that the language deficit of the right-brain-damaged subjects reflects impairment in cognitive structure. Other simultaneous processors such as the formal module (SPLF) that relates linguistic form to the PC are often disrupted as well. This accounts for the deficits right-brain-damaged patients demonstrate when making reference and generating an adequate representation of story structure. When there are any disruptions in the simultaneous processors (PM, CM, SPLF), patients with right-hemisphere damage are less likely to appropriately execute the rules that define pragmatic competence. Preservation of the SCPLF gives these patients control over immediate context and consequently, they are able to construct well-formed sentences. However, problems in accessing aspects of cognitive structure and disruptions in the SPLF limit right-brain-damaged patients' overall ability to construct knowledge or impart their intention to the listener.

This preliminary model attempts to describe the system necessary for implementing and producing discourse. In contrast to the classical left-hemisphere model, this model operates from the assumption that discourse processing involves integrative and mutually dependent processes. This view is consistent with findings suggesting that during discourse production neuroanatomic structures (e.g., Broca's area) do not function in isolation from other parts of the brain. Where a breakdown in a particular aspect of discourse occurred, an adjustment within the language system may be triggered. Both the interaction and dissociation of the components or modules that contribute to discourse production have been considered in an effort to account for the construction of the language system beyond the sentence level.

In conclusion, a model has been presented that could account for bilateral cortical contributions to discourse production. Studies that focus on intrahemispheric localization of lesion are needed to compliment the preliminary observations used to construct the model of discourse production reported here. In addition, the effects of subcortical lesions on discourse must be explored either when they are the primary lesion site, or when they impair discourse by disrupting the behavior of areas to which they connect. Understanding these factors will advance current knowledge of the neurolinguistic system and enrich future models that account for the complexity of discourse processing.

CLINICAL IMPLICATIONS

Two general clinical applications emerge from the research findings and model of discourse production reported here. The first application concerns the identification of communication problems that are only apparent when discourse is considered. Traditionally, assessment of language disorders in adults has focused on the production and comprehension of word and sentence-level stimuli. This method has been appropriate in identifying aspects of aphasic syndromes associated with left-brain damage, but has failed to diagnose less obvious forms of communication impairment in populations such as right-brain-damaged patients. Analysis of discourse has suggested that patients with right-brain damage have difficulty producing the conceptual (Bloom et al., 1992) and pragmatic aspects (Bloom, Borod, Obler, & Gerstman, 1993) of language. These impairments are substantial and remediation for them should be considered.

The second clinical application is based on the proposed model of discourse and its suggestion of how the content, form, and pragmatic aspects of the language system break down following unilateral brain damage. Attention to the interaction of these aspects of discourse provides some potential principles for organizing the assessment and treatment of brain-damaged adults. Both impaired and spared aspects of discourse production should be described when assessing language in patients with brain damage. Further, the model suggests that utilizing a component that is preserved following brain damage may produce a compensation within the language system and promote recovery.

Of particular relevance is the finding that emotional content facilitates pragmatic performance in left-brain-damaged patients (Bloom, Borod, Obler, & Gerstman, 1993). Additional support for this notion comes from experimental studies that have shown that following aphasia emotional content can facilitate performance in auditory comprehension (Reuterskiold, 1991), oral reading (Landis, Graves, & Goodglass, 1982), writing (Landis et al., 1982), and bucco-facial praxis (Borod, Lorch, Koff, & Nicholas, 1987). Certain clinical approaches have been designed to capitalize on preserved functions in aphasia in order to facilitate communication. For example, Visual Action Therapy (Helm-Estabrooks, Fitzpatrick, & Barresi, 1982) uses gestural communication and Melodic Intonation Therapy (Sparks, Helm, & Albert, 1974) utilizes melody that is believed to be a preserved right-hemisphere function. The model proposed in this chapter predicted that recovery in aphasia may be facilitated by procedures that tap into their relatively intact emotional language production capacities. Integrating emotional, social, and linguistic factors into treatment planning may prove to be critical in facilitating recovery from aphasia. Such a treatment approach has recently been described by Lyons (1989).

In right-brain-damaged patients, emotional content suppressed pragmatic performance. Therefore, communication assessment for right-brain damage should consider the negative effects that intrinsically emotional tasks have on language performance. Observation of a patient's personal interactive style in a variety of situations may be necessary to understand the impact of emotional information on communication. Management of right-brain-damaged patients should focus on teaching the use of socially appropriate communication strategies through a hierarchy of emotionally loaded situations (Bloom, Borod, Obler, & Gerstman, 1993). Environmental factors (Lawton, 1991; Lubinski, 1994) and socialization activities (Barr, 1988) should be considered in an effort to create emotionally based clinical contexts that encourage spontaneous communication about real-life events.

In summary, discourse analysis adds clinically significant information that contributes to a better understanding of the linguistic, social, and cognitive status of patients with brain damage. The preliminary model of discourse outlined here suggests that attention should be given to spared and impaired aspects of discourse production. As a clinical tool, discourse analysis has great potential for differentially diagnosing a variety of clinical populations and making predictions about the impact of the language disorder on communication in real-life situations.

REFERENCES

Barr, J. (1988). Group treatment: The logical choice. In B. Shadden (Ed.), *Communication behavior and aging* (pp. 329–340). Baltimore, MD: Williams & Wilkins.

Berko Gleason, J., Goodglass, H., Obler, L., Green, E., Hyde, M., & Weintraub, S. (1980). Narrative strategies of aphasic and normal-speaking subjects. *Journal of Speech and Hearing Research, 23*, 370–382.

Bloom, R., Borod, J., & Obler, L. (1993). *Left and right hemispheric contributions to discourse clarity.* Paper presented at the International Neuropsychological Society, Galveston, TX.

Bloom, R., Borod, J., Obler, L., & Gerstman, L. (1992). Impact of emotional content on discourse production in patients with unilateral brain damage. *Brain and Language, 42*, 153–164.

Bloom, R., Borod, J., Obler, L., & Gerstman, L. (1993). Suppression and facilitation of pragmatic performance: Effects of emotional content on discourse following right and left brain damage. *Journal of Speech and Hearing Research, 36*, 1227–1235.

Borod, J., Lorch, M., Koff, E., & Nicholas, M. (1987). The effect of emotional context on bucco-facial apraxia. *Journal of Clinical and Experimental Neuropsychology, 9*, 147–153.

Buckingham, H. (1982). Neuropsychological models of language. In N. Lass, L. McReynolds, J. Northern, & D. Yoder (Eds.), *Speech, language and hearing* (Vol. I, pp. 323–347). Philadelphia: W. B. Saunders.

Delis, D., Wapner, W., Gardner, H., & Moses, J. (1983). The contribution of the right hemisphere in the organization of paragraphs. *Cortex, 17*, 545–556.

Ernest-Baron, C., Brookshire, R., & Nicholas, L. (1987). Story structure and retelling of narratives by aphasic and non-brain-damaged patients. *Journal of Speech and Hearing Research, 30*, 44–49.

Gardner, H. (1975). *The shattered mind: The person after brain damage.* New York: Alfred A. Knopf.

Gardner, H., Brownell, H., Wapner, W., & Michelow, D. (1983). Missing the point: The role of the right hemisphere in the processing of complex linguistic materials. In E. Perecman (Ed.), *Cognitive processing in the right hemisphere* (pp. 169–189). New York: Academic Press.

Garrett, M. (1980). Levels of processing in sentence production. In B. Butterworth (Ed.), *Language production, Vol. 1: Speech and talk* (pp. 41–64). London: Academic Press.

Helm-Estabrooks, N., Fitzpatrick, P., & Barresi, B. (1982). Visual action therapy for global aphasia. *Journal of Speech and Hearing Disorders, 44*, 385–389.

Huber, W., & Gleber, J. (1982). Linguistic and nonlinguistic processing of narratives in aphasia. *Brain and Language, 16*, 1–18.

Joanette, Y., Goulet, P., Ska, B., & Nespoulous, J. (1986). Informative content of narrative discourse in right brain-damaged right handers. *Brain and Language, 29*, 81–105.

Landis, T., Graves, R., & Goodglass, H. (1982). Aphasic reading and writing: Possible evidence for right hemisphere participation. *Cortex, 18*, 105–112.

Lawton, M. (1991). Older people's uses of the environment in communication. In D. Ripich (Ed.), *Handbook of geriatric communication disorders* (pp. 113–126). Austin, TX: Pro-Ed.

Lubinski, R. (1994). Environmental systems approach to adult aphasia. In R. Chapey (Ed.), *Language intervention strategies in adult aphasia* (pp. 269–291). Baltimore, MD: Williams & Wilkins.

Lyons, J. (1989). Communicative partners: Their value in reestablishing communication with aphasic adults. In T. Prescott (Ed.), *Clinical aphasiology* (Vol. 18, pp. 11–18). Boston: College Hill Press.

Morton, J. (1985). Naming. In S. Epstein & R. Epstein (Eds.), *Current perspectives in dysphasia* (pp. 207–233). Edinburgh: Churchill Livingston.

Perecman, E. (Ed.). (1983). *Cognitive processing in the right hemisphere.* New York: Academic Press.

Reuterskiold, C. (1991). The effects of emotionality on auditory comprehension in aphasia. *Cortex, 27*, 595–604.

Rivers, D., & Love, R. (1980). Language performance on visual processing tasks in right hemisphere lesion cases. *Brain and Language, 10*, 458–466.

Saffran, E. (1982). Neuropsychological approaches to the study of language. *British Journal of Psychology, 73*, 317–337.

Sparks, R., Helm, N., & Albert, M. (1974). Aphasia rehabilitation resulting from Melodic Intonation Therapy. *Cortex, 10*, 303–316.

Ulatowska, H., Freedman-Stern, R., Doyel, A., Macaluso-Haynes, S., & North, A. (1983). Production of narrative discourse in aphasia. *Brain and Language, 19*, 317–334.

Ulatowska, H., North, A., & Macaluso-Haynes, S. (1981). Production of narrative and procedural discourse in aphasia. *Brain and Language, 13*, 345–371.

Walsh, K. (1987). *Neuropsychology: A clinical approach.* New York: Churchill Livingston.

Yorkston, K., & Beukelman, D. (1980). An analysis of connected speech samples of aphasic and normal speakers. *Journal of Speech and Hearing Disorders, 45*, 27–36.

Chapter 6

Cognitive Framework: A Description of Discourse Abilities in Traumatically Brain-Injured Adults

Carl A. Coelho
Gaylord Hospital, Wallingford, CT

Betty Z. Liles
Robert J. Duffy
University of Connecticut, Storrs

The purpose of this chapter is to discuss the application of discourse analyses to the oral verbal communicative behavior of traumatically brain-injured (TBI) adults. We begin with a brief overview of executive functions and the consequent disruption of these processes following TBI. The existing literature on discourse analyses in TBI adults is then reviewed in the context of this model and discussed as evidence of impairments in executive functions.

Traumatic brain injuries are the result of blows to the head and are classified as penetrating (e.g., a gunshot wound) or closed-head (e.g., moving head coming in contact with a stationary object) injuries depending on whether or not the meninges remain intact. Although both closed and penetrating head injuries are classified as TBI, there are distinct differences between the two types, both in terms of array of deficits and recovery, the discussion of which is beyond the scope of this chapter (see Grafman & Salazar, 1987, for a review). For the remainder of this chapter TBI is used to denote individuals who have suffered closed-head injuries only.

IMPAIRMENT OF EXECUTIVE FUNCTIONS FOLLOWING TBI

According to Lezak (1982) "executive functions comprise those mental capacities necessary for formulating goals, planning how to achieve them, and carrying out the plans effectively" (p. 281). Executive function does not represent a discrete process but rather an umbrella function that comes into play with all realms of cognitive processing. When executive function is impaired, all other cognitive systems (e.g., attention, memory, reasoning, etc.) have the potential to be affected even though they may individually remain intact (Sohlberg & Mateer, 1989). Sohlberg and Mateer have noted that damage to the frontal lobes results in behavioral and emotional deficits as well as cognitive deficits, particularly decreased executive function. According to Stuss and Benson (1986), the frontal lobes coordinate input from all other regions of the brain and therefore are important for coordinating and actualizing activities involved in cognitive processing. However, Goldberg and Bilder (1987) argued that prefrontal pathology is not necessary to produce "executive syndrome" and that this syndrome may be relatively common in any diffuse brain dysfunction.

Ylvisaker and Szekeres (1989) noted that following severe TBI most individuals demonstrate communicative deficits directly attributable to disruption of executive functions. They list seven broad dimensions of executive function in which this dysfunction may occur:

1. Self-awareness and goal setting: involving decreased insight of cognitive and verbal deficits as well as the implications of such deficits.
2. Planning: involving decreased knowledge of the appropriate steps to complete a task and/or the ability to sequence and organize these steps.
3. Self-directing/initiating: involving a decreased ability to initiate an activity, despite having all of the necessary resources, without prompting from another individual.
4. Self-inhibiting: involving an impaired ability to inhibit verbal behavior that may be impulsive, tangential, perseverative, or socially inappropriate.
5. Self-monitoring: involving decreased monitoring of the context (social or otherwise) that a behavior occurs in.
6. Self-evaluation: involving a decreased ability to evaluate performance objectively.
7. Flexible problem solving: involving an impaired ability to revise a plan and consider alternative solutions when presented with new information.

This framework is applied to the discourse deficits that have been noted in adults with TBI. Prior to that discussion however, an overview of these discourse deficits is presented.

IMPAIRMENTS OF DISCOURSE ABILITIES FOLLOWING TBI

A variety of investigations has examined discourse abilities of TBI adults. These studies have analyzed discourse skills at the levels of story structure, intersentential cohesion and cohesive adequacy, and conversation. Initially, the principal findings from three studies most relevant to story structure and cohesion are summarized by level of analysis. Studies related to the analysis of conversation are also reviewed as appropriate.

Prior to reviewing the findings on story structure and cohesion, information relating to subject characteristics, discourse elicitation tasks, and analyses from these three studies are presented.

Subject Characteristics. In each of the three studies adults with closed-head injuries were studied (11 by Hartley & Jensen, 1991; 3 by Mentis & Prutting, 1987; and 4 by Liles, Coelho, Duffy, & Zalagens, 1989). Liles et al.'s subjects were selected for study because they had recovered a high level of functional language; that is, they all evidenced fluent discourse and did not demonstrate any significant deficits on traditional clinical language tests. With regard to the TBI subjects' motor speech deficits, Hartley and Jensen noted that 7 of their 11 subjects had either a mild or moderate dysarthria, Mentis and Prutting reported that 2 of their 3 subjects were dysarthric, and none of Liles et al.'s subjects were dysarthric.

In all three studies, the discourse performances of the TBI subjects were compared to those of a group of normal controls (Hartley and Jensen's group consisted of 21, Mentis and Prutting 3, and Liles et al., 23). In the Liles et al. study, the scores of the TBI subjects were converted to z scores for the purpose of comparing them to the average performance of normal subjects. Z scores of the TBI subjects that fell within the range of +1.65 to −1.65 were considered to be within normal limits (a z value greater than 1.65 represents the upper and lower 5% of a normal distribution of the normal subjects).

Discourse Elicitation and Analysis Procedures. In each of the three studies different narrative elicitation tasks and analysis procedures were employed. Hartley and Jensen employed story generation (telling a story based on a comic strip), story retelling (retelling a story presented auditorily), and procedural discourse (telling how to buy groceries) tasks. Units of measure included productivity, content, and cohesion. Mentis and Prutting presented their subjects with two discourse tasks: conversational (10 minutes of unstructured conversation) and narrative (three tasks: description of work or therapy program the subject was participating in, telling how to play a favorite sport, and telling how to bake a cake or change a tire). Cohesion analysis followed Halliday and Hasan's (1976, 1989) procedure with the number and type of each cohesive tie identified. Liles et al. elicited stories from their subjects under two conditions: retelling and generation. In the retelling condition, subjects were shown a film strip picture story and instructed to retell the story. In the generation condition, subjects were shown a copy of a picture and instructed to tell a story about what they felt was happening (while the picture remained in view). Measurement of story narrative performance was made at three levels: sentence production, intersentential cohesion, and story structure.

Story Structure

Story structure knowledge refers to the purported regularities in the internal structure of stories that guide an individual's comprehension and production of the logical relationships between people and events (e.g., temporal and causal). Descriptions of story structures differ, but the episode unit is central to virtually all models proposed by recent investigators (Frederiksen, 1975; Johnson & Mandler, 1980; Meyer, 1975; Rumelhart, 1975; Stein & Glenn, 1979; Thorndyke, 1977; Thorndyke & Yekovitch, 1980). Because the relationships among components of the episode are considered to be logical and not bound by specific content, researchers describe episode organization as being in the cognitive domain. The episode components are defined as units (i.e., statements) bearing information about stated goals, attempts at solutions, and the consequences of these attempts. Stein and Glenn (1979) identified these components as initiating event, attempt, and direct consequence. The creation of episodes is evidence of story structure knowledge, and because this unit is cognitive in nature it is reasonable to believe that it may be disrupted by damage to the brain.

Liles et al. were the only investigators to employ story structure analysis. Findings from that study indicated that TBI and normal subjects produced a comparable number of episodes in story retelling. In story generation, however, three of the four TBI subjects produced no episodes. The stimulus picture used for story generation depicted three characters in a specific context at one point in time. Adequate story development would depend on the speaker's ability to transpose a static representation of the events (i.e., the picture) to a dynamic representation (i.e., story development). Blank, Rose, and Berlin (1978) referred to such a disparity between the context and required language use a cognitive "re-ordering." The TBI subjects' inability to use episode structure in the story-generation task, in spite of having been able to generate complete episodes in the story-retelling task, suggests that the interaction of cognition and language required of the generation task was extremely difficult for them.

Intersentential Cohesion

Cohesion is defined as structural coherence among parts of a text (Halliday & Hasan, 1976, 1989). Sentences are conjoined by various kinds of meaning relations described as cohesive ties. The kinds of ties vary, depending on the nature of the text (i.e., communicative function), the style and ability of the speaker. A speaker's relative frequency of use of the various categories of cohesive ties is referred to as *cohesive style* (Liles et al., 1989). Each of the different types of discourse (e.g., procedural, descriptive, story narratives, conversational) is distinct and therefore, requires a different pattern of cohesive use to instantiate the underlying rules of structure appropriate to the creation of coherent text. Speakers normally shift their patterns of cohesive use across types of discourse; they may also modify cohesive use in response to differences in the context in which the text is being created. Analysis of intersentential cohesion may involve the frequency of occurrence of, for example, Halliday and Hasan's five cohesive categories: reference, lexical, conjunctive, ellipsis, and substitution (see Liles et al., 1989, and Mentis & Prutting, 1987, for definitions of these categories).

Hartley and Jensen (1991) found that TBI patients produced fewer cohesive ties per utterance than did normal speakers in both narrative and procedural discourse. Mentis and Prutting (1987) also noted that their TBI subjects used fewer cohesive ties than the normal subjects in narrative tasks. These findings are in contrast to those of Liles et al. (1989), who noted that the number of cohesive ties (per T-unit) produced by their TBI subjects was the same as the normal controls for both story generation and story retelling. Differences in the proportional use of cohesive ties across discourse tasks were reported in both the Mentis and Prutting and Liles et al. studies. Mentis and Prutting stated that the use of different cohesion patterns by the TBI subjects appeared to be related to their reduced linguistic processing abilities, their limited pragmatic abilities, and their attempts at compensating for linguistic deficits. Liles et al. reported that in a story-retelling task similar proportions of referential, lexical, and conjunctive markers occurred in both subject groups. However, in story generation a major difference between the groups emerged in which the TBI subjects showed a striking reversal of the pattern of the normal subjects as well as a reversal of their own cohesive pattern used in the story-retelling task. In story generation all of the TBI subjects decreased the proportional use of reference and increased the proportion of lexical ties. Liles et al. attributed this finding to the TBI subjects' apparent direct reference to the stimulus picture. These direct references were characterized as interjected descriptors of the picture that were unrelated to the rest of the text. The authors further stated that the TBI subjects rarely integrated these lexical items into the text structure and consequently such items were often judged to be incomplete ties. The TBI subjects' rather marked tendency to refer outside their texts suggests that they were unable to detach themselves from the perceptual salience of the picture in order to organize their language for story development. Blank et al.'s (1978) notion of cognitive reordering, previously discussed in the section on story structure, is applicable to these findings as well. This explanation further suggests that the TBI subjects could not consistently engage in the interaction of cognition and language use that was required in the story-generation task.

Cohesive Adequacy

Each occurrence of a cohesive marker (i.e., tie) is also judged as to its adequacy. For example, using Liles' (1985) procedure, three categories of adequacy are possible: (a) a tie is judged "complete" if the information referred to by the cohesive marker is easily found and defined with no ambiguity, (b) a tie is judged "incomplete" if the information referred to by the cohesive marker was not provided in the text, and (c) a tie is judged to be an "error" if the listener was guided to ambiguous information elsewhere in the text.

Mentis and Prutting noted that their TBI subjects used incomplete ties, which was not characteristic of the normal subjects. Liles et al. observed that like the normal subjects, the TBI subjects showed greater cohesive adequacy in the story-retelling task, in which they demonstrated a higher percentage of complete ties and a lower percentage of incomplete ties than in the story-generation task. However, in the story-generation task, two of the four TBI subjects exhibited a much lower percentage of complete ties than normal subjects. Error ties were rare in both groups of subjects.

Longitudinal Assessment of Cohesion and Story Grammar

In the three studies just reviewed, TBI subjects' discourse abilities and intersentential cohesion and story grammar in particular, were sampled on single occasions. To date, only one investigation has examined discourse performances of TBI subjects sampled longitudinally. Over a period of several months, Coelho, Liles, and Duffy (1991a) collected discourse samples from two individuals with TBI. These subjects were selected for study because of their functional language skills and fluent discourse.

Discourse samples were elicited with a story-generation task. Subjects were shown a copy of a Norman Rockwell painting and instructed to tell a story about what was happening in the picture. This procedure was repeated every 2 weeks and eventually on a monthly basis. Stories were analyzed at the levels of intersentential cohesion and story grammar.

Each subject demonstrated a distinct profile of discourse abilities and each profile was associated with a different pattern of recovery. The scores of the TBI subjects were converted to *z* scores for the purpose of comparing them to the average performance of the control subjects. The control subjects were 23 college sophomores (ages 18–22 years) with no history of neurologic disease or trauma (a control group made up of college students was felt to be appropriate as both TBI subjects were in their early 20s and either a college graduate or in college at the time of their injury).

Subject 1's stories were characterized by poorly organized sentences, as reflected by her intersentential cohesion scores. The number of complete ties per T-unit was consistently below the mean of the normal subjects in the story generation task. In spite of Subject 1's poorly organized narratives, the content was task appropriate. The number of complete episodes approached and eventually surpassed the mean for the control subjects on this task (see Fig. 6.1). Although Subject 1's early narratives did contain complete episodes, the narratives also contained information that had little or no relevance to her story.

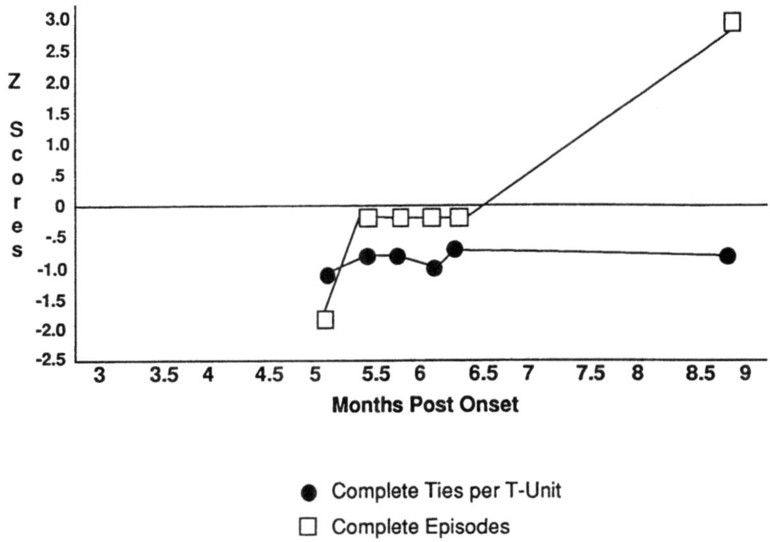

FIG. 6.1. Number of complete ties per T-unit and complete episodes plotted over time for Subject 1. (From Coelho, Liles, & Duffy, 1991a. Reprinted by permission of W. B. Saunders.)

The examiners concluded that the subject was inserting idiosyncratic associations and did not appear to be able to make plausible judgments about how to integrate this information into the context as presented in the picture. Her lack of development of these associations resulted in numerous cohesive references with no semantic ties to other parts of the text.

Subject 2's discourse performance assessed with the same measures and elicitation task represented a second distinct profile. In contrast to Subject 1, Subject 2's stories were cohesively well organized (i.e., meaning was tied across sentences). The number of complete ties per T-unit for the story-generation task was below the normal subjects' mean performance but did improve over time. As can be seen in the number of complete episodes, the content of Subject 2's stories was poor. This subject never produced a complete episode in this story-generation task (see Fig. 6.2).

Prognostically, Subject 1 was felt to be less significantly impaired than Subject 2. The presence of appropriate, albeit disorganized, content was an early indication that Subject 1 was attaching some meaning to the stimuli from the elicitation task, and that she was able to appreciate the potential relationships/roles of the characters who appeared in the Rockwell picture. As recovery occurred, Subject 1's improvement was reflected in her development and integration of the tangential associations, the organization of the content of her stories, and the number of complete episodes.

Subject 2 demonstrated a far more severe pattern of cognitive dysfunction. Her attempts at stories were merely elaborate descriptions of the picture used

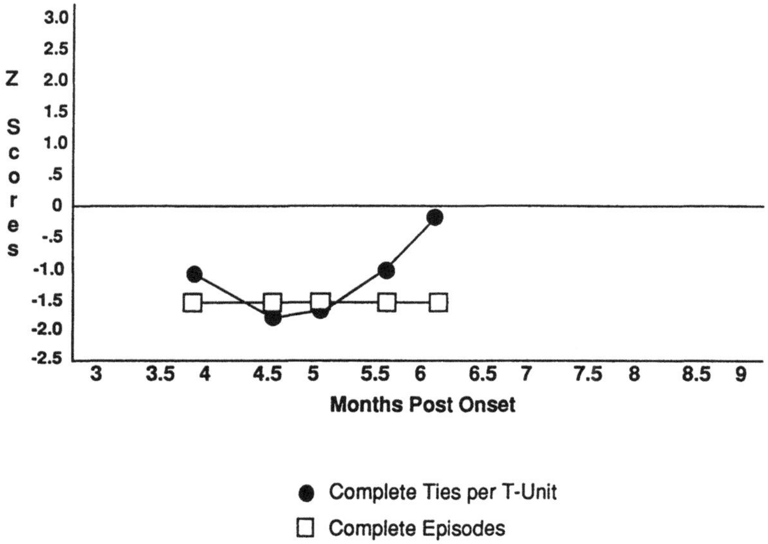

FIG. 6.2. Number of complete ties per T-unit and complete episodes plotted over time for Subject 2. (From Coelho, Liles, & Duffy, 1991a. Reprinted by permission of W. B. Saunders.)

for the generation task. She never demonstrated any appreciation of the relationships among the characters, and appeared unable to detach herself from that moment in time, represented in the picture, to generate episodes regarding why the characters were together or what might happen next. Organization of her utterances was good, but the content was lacking.

This procedure appeared to have ecologic validity in that Subject 1, the least impaired as measured by this procedure, was eventually able to return to competitive employment and to work productively. Subject 2, who was clearly more impaired, not only experienced difficulty with coursework when she returned to school, but reportedly had significant problems maintaining relationships with fellow students.

Conversation

A number of recent investigations of the discourse abilities of individuals with TBI have focused on conversational discourse (Coelho, Liles, & Duffy, 1991b; Coelho, Liles, Duffy, & Clarkson, 1993; Ehrlich & Sipes, 1985; Mentis & Prutting, 1991; Penn & Cleary, 1988). Interest in this discourse form has arisen from the contention that the assessment of communicative skills in higher level head-injured adults may be facilitated by the use of functionally oriented tasks (Milton, 1988). Conversational discourse, which more closely approximates the social-interactional nature of communication, is an example of such tasks. Further,

Ehrlich and Sipes (1985) emphasized that not only should such tasks be assessed but they should become a focus of treatment as well. Published reports on the analysis of conversational discourse have examined a variety of analysis categories including utterance appropriateness, topic maintenance, and compensatory strategies. Each of these general categories of analysis is reviewed here.

Appropriateness of an Utterance. Blank and Franklin (1980) described a procedure for evaluating the appropriateness of an utterance within a conversation. The concept of appropriateness has received some attention in the psychiatric literature because its absence is seen as an important element in the interpersonal difficulties of both neurotic and psychotic individuals. However, this issue has not traditionally been addressed objectively in the assessment of brain-injured individuals. Using the distinction of speaker-initiator and speaker-responder, appropriateness within a conversational interchange can be examined. The utterances of the speaker-initiator are evaluated according to what Blank and Franklin termed their *summoning power*. Utterances that clearly summon or demand a response are designated as *obliges*, whereas those that do not are designated as *comments*. A differential response to these conversational initiatives describes whether the speaker is appropriately extending the conversation. The quality of the speaker-responder's utterances is evaluated on a scale of appropriateness (adequate+, adequate, inadequate, ambiguous).

Coelho et al. (1991b) applied this analysis procedure to the conversational discourse of five TBI and five normal subjects engaged in conversations with the same research assistant. Results indicated that the two groups could be distinguished on the basis of (a) the TBI subjects' greater number of turns per conversation, (b) the research assistant's higher percentage of oblige production in conversations with the TBI subjects, and (c) the quality of the speakers' responses. Within each 15-minute conversation both the subject and the research assistant functioned as an initiator and a responder. Turns, therefore, accounted for all utterances produced by each participant in a conversation. The greater number of turns in the TBI subjects' conversations was attributable to a number of factors, including their shorter length of utterance per turn and the research assistant's high percentage of obliges. It appeared as though the TBI subjects had more difficulty initiating and sustaining conversations than the normal controls. The research assistant attempted to compensate for this by using more obliges in an effort to draw the TBI subjects into dialogue. Furthermore, the TBI subjects' decreased ability to extend connected discourse (i.e., lower frequency and adequacy of their responses) with the research assistant resulted in dialogue containing utterances that were at times disjointed and seemingly irrelevant to the conversation. Thus, some of the information expressed by the TBI subjects required interpretation and clarification, which in turn generated additional obliges (questions) from the research assistant for complete understanding. With regard to the quality of the speakers' responses, normal controls' greater production of adequate+ responses (responses that relevantly elaborated the theme so as to provide more information than was requested) was also consistent with their lower number of turns per conversation. The normal subjects, as well as the research assistant when she was conversing with them, were more likely to develop and extend dialogue on specific topics as opposed to the shorter, less elaborated discussions that took place with the TBI subjects.

Topic Initiation and Maintenance. How individuals manage conversational topics is critical to the success of an interaction. *Topic* refers to what conversations are about and how what they are about changes as an interaction proceeds (Brinton & Fujiki, 1989). Initiation of a new topic is often marked only by the introduction of propositional content (Hurtig, 1977); in other words, a speaker simply begins talking about something else. Sometimes speakers initiate new topics by using special devices such as an opening marker (e.g., "By the way . . .") or questions that signal the listener that the topic is changing. After a topic is initiated in conversation, it may or may not be continued in the utterances that follow. A topic is said to be "maintained" when it is continued (Brinton & Fujiki, 1989). Although a topic may be maintained by a single speaker, in conversational dyads topics are maintained by both participants. Topics may be discontinued when the speakers stop talking or when the speakers change topics. Topics may also be discontinued and a new topic initiated subtly, which is referred to as *topic shading* (Brinton & Fujiki, 1989). Such topic shifts may be smooth or disruptive.

Coelho et al. (1991) examined the manner of topic initiation of 5 TBI, 5 mildly aphasic (3 nonfluent and 2 fluent), and 5 normal subjects during 15 minutes of conversation. Topics could be introduced by either a subject or their conversational partner (which was the same research assistant for all 15 subjects). Topics could be changed in three ways: (a) at the beginning of the conversation, or by ending discussion of one topic and initiating another, referred to as *novel introduction*; (b) by means of a *smooth shift*, in which discussion of one topic is subtly switched to another; or (c) by means of a *disruptive shift*, in which discussion of one topic is abruptly or illogically switched to another topic. Results indicated that the normal controls initiated 59% of all topics in their conversations with the research assistant. This was in marked contrast to the TBI subjects who introduced 28% and the aphasic subjects who introduced 20% of all topics in their conversations with the research assistant. With regard to manner of topic initiation, in the conversational dyads with the normals and the research assistant, nearly equal numbers of novel introductions were noted, 1.4 and 1.2, respectively. The TBI subjects had a mean of only .2 novel introductions, whereas the research assistant had a mean of 1.6 in his or her conversations. In the conversations with the aphasic subjects and the research assistant, only the research assistant had novel introductions, with a mean of 4.4. All subjects had comparable mean numbers of smooth shifts, 3.2 for the normal controls and 2.6 for the TBI and aphasic subjects. The research assistant had the smallest mean number of smooth shifts in the conversations with the normal controls (1.8), a larger mean number in the conversations with the TBI subjects (6.8), and the greatest mean number with the aphasic subjects (8.8). Disruptive shifts accounted for very few of the topic changes in any of the conversational dyads.

Overall, the TBI and aphasic subjects had more difficulty initiating and sustaining conversations than did the normal controls as indicated by the low number of topic initiations by both brain-injured groups of subjects. The research assistant attempted to compensate for this by using more obliges, changing topics within the conversation, and doing more talking (i.e., the research assistant produced a greater proportion of the total words in the conversations with the TBI and aphasic subjects than in those with the normal controls). In examining the content within the research assistant's obliges across groups it appeared that the research assistant used obliges for different reasons with each of the brain-injured groups. For example, the research assistant made more requests for clarification of the aphasic subjects, possibly due to their high proportion of agrammatic utterances. With the TBI subjects, obliges were used to elicit more content on a specific topic or to change topics when the conversation lagged.

Mentis and Prutting (1991) developed a multidimensional analysis procedure for delineating patterns and problems in topic management. Analysis parameters included such items as type and manner of topic introduction, intonation units, side sequence units, and problematic ideational units. Six conversational and four monologue samples of a TBI adult and a matched normal adult were compared using this analysis procedure. Results indicated that the TBI subject demonstrated disrupted topic management abilities as seen in the subject's production of (a) noncoherent topic changes; (b) ambiguous, unrelated, and incomplete ideational units; and (c) unrelated issues. These features resulted in a decrease in overall textual coherence and continuity of topic development. The authors noted that the reduction in the TBI subject's topic management abilities resulted in a greater reliance on the structure provided for him by his conversational partner than did the normal subject. This observation is consistent with the findings of Coelho et al. (1993).

Compensatory Strategies. The compensatory strategies employed by six individuals with TBI in conversational discourse have been described by Penn and Cleary (1988). Strategy types were classified into seven categories: simplification, elaboration, repetition, fluency, sociolinguistic, nonverbal, and interlocutor. Results indicated that all subjects made use of a wide range of strategies in an attempt to compensate for both cognitive and language deficits, with differential effectiveness. The authors stated that it was unclear why certain subjects adopted certain strategies; however, it was most likely due to a combination of factors including severity of deficits, age, time post onset, plus the influence of therapy and environmental context.

DISCOURSE DEFICITS AS EVIDENCE OF IMPAIRMENT IN EXECUTIVE FUNCTIONS

Based on this review, it is evident that individuals with TBI demonstrate an array of discourse deficits. These deficits are demonstrated in a variety of discourse forms and analyses. Coelho, Liles, and Duffy (in press), using a story-retelling task, monitored discourse performance in a mildly aphasic individual (secondary to a single unilateral left thrombo-embolic CVA) over a period of 12 months and noted that as severity of aphasia decreased (as measured by the Porch, 1981, Index of Communicative Ability) sentence formulation and cohesion abilities improved. Story structure abilities, however, remained relatively impaired. This finding would appear to be inconsistent with those of previous investigators who noted that even in moderately impaired aphasic individuals, essential elements of superstructure (defined as categories of story structure—setting, action, resolution, and evaluation—or as steps of instrumental scripts—e.g., steps required for changing a light bulb) are well preserved (Ulatowska, Freedman-Stern, Weiss-Doyel, Macaluso-Haynes, & North, 1983; Ulatowska, North, & Macaluso-Haynes, 1981; Ulatowska, Weiss-Doyel, Freedman-Stern, Macaluso-Haynes, & North, 1983). However, it should be noted that these studies employed elicitation tasks requiring descriptions of action sequences or procedures that may not have tapped story structure abilities. Further, the mildly aphasic subject studied by Coelho et al. did exhibit rudimentary story structures in all of his story retellings, but over the 12-month period that his discourse performance was monitored, story structure ability did not improve or recover to the degree that his sentence formulation and cohesion abilities did. This discrepancy suggests that story structure ability may be more cognitively based than linguistic. The authors further noted that story structure dysfunction may be a result of brain injury in general versus simply aphasia.

This notion is consistent with the clinical observation that in the face of functional performance on standardized language batteries and good sentence-level grammar, the communicative abilities of adults with TBI are frequently judged to be inadequate (Coelho et al., 1991a; Holland, 1982; Liles et al., 1989). The discourse deficits reviewed here serve as a partial explanation for the observed pragmatic-communicative deficiencies. However, these impairments in discourse performance may be considered secondary deficits and merely a reflection of a more global primary impairment of executive function. Lezak (1983) observed that the executive function system can "break down at any stage in the behavioral sequence that makes up planned or intentional activity" (p. 508). Using Ylvisaker and Szekeres' (1989) framework of communicative deficits attributable to disruption of executive function, previously described, we interpret the findings from the studies on discourse performances of TBI subjects in terms of impaired executive function.

Story Structure

Adequate production and comprehension of a story depends on the logical sequence of cognitively based story structures. These structures guide an individual's interpretations, expectations, and inferences about the possible relationships between people and events in a story. The very nature of an episode is consistent with executive functions. Episodes form a framework for stories organizing content as behavioral sequences consisting of three parts: (a) an initiating event causing a character to formulate a goal-directed sequence, (b) an action, and (c) a direct consequence marking attainment or nonattainment of the goal. Episode generation requires identification of goals, recognition of an intended plan, and evaluation of the success or failure of this plan with regard to attainment of the goal.

The TBI subjects studied demonstrated difficulty formulating episodes in the story-generation task. Although they were able to recall complete episodes from the stimulus filmstrip in the story-retelling task they were unable to use episode structure for story generation.

This disparity in the subjects' performance across the retelling and generation tasks may be interpreted to mean that executive planning was not required in the retelling task to the same extent as in the generation task because of the structured presentation of the pictured story. In contrast, the story-generation task required the subjects to internalize, or enter into the world of the story in space and time, and reorganize the pictured scene into a logical and coherent structure.

Cohesion and Cohesive Adequacy

The notion of cohesiveness refers to the organization and clarity of a narrative text. Cohesive ties conjoin sentences by various kinds of meaning relations. Adequate cohesion may require an individual to analyze the content of a proposed narrative and to select a structure or format of organization (cohesive pattern) to best instantiate the intended meaning. More specifically, the individual is required to make choices about what kinds of linguistic devices should be used to coordinate the meaning across sentences. These choices are made in light of the text's function (e.g., procedures, story, etc.) and structure (e.g., causal and temporal organization of content). This process would implicate goal formulation, planning (i.e., sequencing and organization), self-monitoring and problem solving (to monitor the relationship between task requirements and content and to be able to make the appropriate adjustments in the cohesive pattern). Clearly, dimensions of executive function are critical for the adequate use of cohesion.

The principal findings related to cohesion and cohesive adequacy were that the TBI subjects produced a lower percentage of complete ties in their narratives on certain tasks. In addition, there were differences noted in the proportional use of certain types of cohesive ties across tasks. Specifically, in story generation because the TBI subjects were apparently unable to detach themselves from the perceptual salience of the stimulus picture, they were unable to integrate language for story development. Therefore, a decrease in the proportional use of reference and an increase in the use of lexical ties was noted. Although cohesion interacts with episode organization, because both episodes and local sentences' coherence must be considered, the systems can be distinguished. A speaker may, under some circumstances, produce a coherent rendition if the content is very simple or overlearned (e.g., the story-retelling task). One may propose then at some level of an overlearned task, intersentential cohesion would require little executive planning.

Conversation

Brinton and Fujiki (1989) observed that "the ability to participate in conversation is basic to getting along from day to day in society" (p. 1). Conversation is a dynamic and complex activity that requires participants to adhere to certain rules as they interact. Management of these rules for turn taking, topic initiation and maintenance, and conversational repair determines both the quality and success of a conversation. Meaningful participation in conversations requires that each participant have an ongoing awareness of his or her partner's perspective or needs, be able to initiate and change topics throughout the interaction, to inhibit comments or other behaviors that are inappropriate to the exchange, and to continually monitor the overall flow of the conversation and make necessary adjustments as needed. Executive functions are obviously critical to successful conversational performance.

TBI subjects, as mentioned earlier, demonstrated difficulty initiating and sustaining conversations as illustrated by their shorter turns, the limited number of topics they introduced in conversations, and the shorter less elaborated discussions that occurred in their conversations. Further, the TBI subjects were reliant on their conversational partner to maintain the flow of the conversation seen in part in the high proportion of oblige production by the partner. When TBI subjects did introduce topics it was as times at the expense of textual coherence and continuity of overall topic development. Finally, although TBI subjects attempted to compensate for difficulty in conversational interactions, the strategies employed were not always effective.

IMPLICATIONS

Although the interpretation of discourse deficits as an impairment of executive functions is logically very appealing, a great deal of research remains to be done related to the development of this explanation. Investigation of the potential relationships between measures of cognitive abilities (e.g., attention and memory) and measures of discourse performance (e.g., story structure, cohesion, topic maintenance) would be an important beginning. Development of a model depicting the hypothesized relationship of discourse abilities to executive function should also be undertaken and eventually tested. In any event, this explanation has great potential with regard to its clinical implications. From the perspective of assessing executive functions, which is frequently difficult because the nature of formal testing often compensates for many of the dimensions of executive function examiners seek to measure (Lezak, 1982), discourse measures may provide a means of objectifying deficits of executive function in natural, everyday communicative behaviors and environments. From the perspective of assessing and treating discourse impairments, this explanation provides a better understanding of the functional consequences of such deficits. In other words, discourse deficits may be indicative of significant, and functionally more compromising, impairments than simply an inability to tell a story. Finally, the study of the relationship between executive function and discourse abilities can shed light on the nature of the cognitive and language impairments of individuals with TBI.

REFERENCES

Blank, M., & Franklin, E. (1980). Dialogue with preschoolers: A cognitively-based system of assessment. *Applied Psycholinguistics, 1*, 127–150.

Blank, M., Rose, S. A., & Berlin, L. J. (1978). *Preschool language assessment instrument: The assessment of learning in practice.* New York: Grune & Stratton.

Brinton, B., & Fujiki, M. (1989). *Conversational management with language-impaired children.* Rockville, MD: Aspen.

Coelho, C. A., Liles, B. Z., & Duffy, R. J. (1991a). Discourse analyses with closed head injured adults: Evidence for differing patterns of deficits. *Archives of Physical Medicine and Rehabilitation, 72*, 465–468.

Coelho, C. A., Liles, B. Z., & Duffy, R. J. (1991b). Analysis of conversational discourse in head-injured adults. *Journal of Head Trauma Rehabilitation, 6*, 92–99.

Coelho, C. A., Liles, B. Z., & Duffy, R. J. (in press). Longitudinal assessment of narrative discourse in a mildly aphasic adult. *Clinical Aphasiology.*

Coelho, C. A., Liles, B. Z., Duffy, R. J., & Clarkson, J. V. (1993). Conversational patterns of aphasic, closed head injured, and normal speakers. *Clinical Aphasiology, 21*, 183–192.

Ehrlich, J. S., & Sipes, A. L. (1985). Group treatment of communication skills for head trauma patients. *Cognitive Rehabilitation, 3*, 32–37.

Frederiksen, C. H. (1975). Representing logical and semantic structures of knowledge acquired from discourse. *Cognitive Psychology, 7*, 371–458.

Goldberg, E., & Bilder, R. M. (1987). The frontal lobes and hierarchical organization of cognitive control. In E. Perecman (Ed.), *The frontal lobes revisited* (pp. 159–187). New York: IRBN Press.

Grafman, J., & Salazar, A. (1987). Methodological considerations relevant to the comparison of recovery from penetrating and closed head injuries. In H. Levin, J. Grafman, & H. Eisenberg (Eds.), *Neurobehavioral recovery from head injury* (pp. 43–54). New York: Oxford University Press.

Halliday, M. A. K., & Hasan, R. (1976). *Cohesion in English.* London: Longman Group.

Halliday, M. A. K., & Hasan, R. (1989). *Language, context & text: Aspects of language in a social-semiotic perspective.* New York: Oxford University Press.

Hartley, L., & Jensen, P. J. (1991). Narrative and procedural discourse after closed head injury. *Brain Injury, 5*, 267.

Holland, A. (1982). When is aphasia aphasia? The problem with closed head injury. *Clinical Aphasiology, 12*, 345–349.

Hurtig, R. (1977). Toward a functional theory of discourse. In R. O. Freedle (Ed.), *Discourse production and comprehension* (pp. 89–106). Norwood, NJ: Ablex.

Johnson, N. S., & Mandler, J. M. (1980). A tale of two structures: Underlying and surface forms in stories. *Poetics, 9*, 51–86.

Lezak, M. (1982). The problem of assessing executive functions. *International Journal of Psychology, 17*, 281–297.

Lezak, M. (1983). *Neuropsychological assessment.* New York: Oxford University Press.

Liles, B. Z. (1985). Narrative ability in normal and language-disordered children. *Journal of Speech and Hearing Research, 23*, 123–133.

Liles, B. Z., Coelho, C. A., Duffy, R. J., & Zalagens, M. (1989). Effects of elicitation procedures on the narratives of normal and closed head-injured adults. *Journal of Speech and Hearing Disorders, 54*, 356–366.

Mentis, M., & Prutting, C. A. (1987). Cohesion in the discourse of normal and head-injured adults. *Journal of Speech and Hearing Research, 30*, 88–98.

Mentis, M., & Prutting, C. A. (1991). Analysis of topic as illustrated in a head-injured and a normal adult. *Journal of Speech and Hearing Research, 34*, 583–595.

Meyer, B. J. F. (1975). Identification of the structure of prose and its implications for the study of reading and memory. *Journal of Reading Behavior, 7*, 7–47.

Milton, S. B. (1988). Management of subtle cognitive communication deficits. *Journal of Head Trauma Rehabilitation, 3*, 1–11.

Penn, C., & Cleary, J. (1988). Compensatory strategies in the language of closed head injured patients. *Brain Injury, 2*, 3–17.

Porch, B. E. (1981). *Porch Index of Communicative Ability.* Palo Alto, CA: Consulting Psychologists Press.

Rumelhart, D. E. (1975). Notes on a schema for stories. In D. G. Bobrow & A. M. Collins (Eds.), *Representation and understanding: Studies in cognitive science* (pp. 211–236). Hillsdale, NJ: Lawrence Erlbaum Associates.

Sohlberg, M. M., & Mateer, C. A. (1989). *Introduction to cognitive rehabilitation theory and practice.* New York: Guilford Press.

Stein, N. L., & Glenn, C. G. (1979). An analysis of story comprehension in elementary school children. In R. O. Freedle (Ed.), *New directions in discourse processing* (Vol. 2, pp. 53–120). Norwood, NJ: Ablex.

Stuss, D., & Benson, F. (1986). *The frontal lobes.* New York: Raven Press.

Thorndyke, P. W. (1977). Cognitive structures in comprehension and memory of narrative discourse. *Cognitive Psychology, 9*, 77–100.

Thorndyke, P. W., & Yekovitch, F. R. (1980). A critique of schemata as a theory of human story memory. *Poetics, 9*, 23–49.

Ulatowska, H. K., Freedman-Stern, R., Weiss-Doyel, A., Macaluso-Haynes, S., & North, A. J. (1983). Production of narrative discourse in aphasia. *Brain and Language, 19*, 317–334.

Ulatowska, H. K., North, A. J., & Macaluso-Haynes, S. (1981). Production of narrative and procedural discourse in aphasia. *Brain and Language, 13*, 345–371.

Ulatowska, H. K., Weiss-Doyel, A., Freedman-Stern, R., Macaluso-Haynes, S. M., & North, A. J. (1983). Production of procedural discourse in aphasia. *Brain and Language, 18*, 315–341.

Ylvisaker, M., & Szekeres, S. F. (1989). Metacognitive and executive impairments in head-injured children and adults. *Topics in Language Disorders, 9*, 34–49.

Chapter 7

The Expression of Pragmatic Intentions in Adults With Mental Retardation During Instructional Discourse

Robert A. Domingo
Long Island University/C.W. Post Campus

The communicative abilities of adults with mental retardation have long been the subject of considerable investigation. Although early research in the area of their speech and language (Blount, 1968; Schiefelbusch, 1972) focused more on characterizing phonological and grammatical aspects, recently this approach has been replaced by a more "functional" orientation. *Functional communication skills* are defined as those skills that are "useful to the adult in terms of meeting his/her environmental and communicative demands" (Bedrosian, 1988, p. 266).

This change in research orientation grew naturally out of an awareness that knowledge of grammar is only part of what speakers need to know about their native language; that in order to use language appropriately for communicative purposes, speakers must also possess knowledge of a system of rules and conventions for using language in various settings and with different interlocutors. The new research, developed from a sociolinguistic framework, emphasizes the importance of examining interactive abilities and social skills within naturally occurring contexts (Anderson-Levitt & Platt, 1984; Graffam, 1983; Kernan & Sabsay, 1982, 1987; Linder, 1978a, 1978b; Platt, 1984; Turner, 1982).

This chapter introduces one such naturally occurring context—the adult day treatment program. In this program, instructional discourse is constructed between program participants and teaching staff. The chapter also examines the ability of program participants to self-regulate or "control" different instructional interactions through the use of dominant or submissive utterances. This ability to *self-regulate* or *control* refers to the (proposed) innate ability one has to monitor his or her own language in an interaction to avoid communicative breakdowns (e.g., to know when to re-formulate when one perceives that a message has not been adequately delivered; Schegloff, Jefferson, & Sacks, 1977).

In order to best understand the discourse analysis that follows, it is first necessary to describe the communicative context in question (i.e., the adult day treatment program).

THE ADULT DAY TREATMENT PROGRAM

Once young people with mental retardation grow too old for continued special educational placements, those deemed not ready for joining the work force in the community may find themselves placed in day treatment programs. These programs are designed to aid in the development of greater independence and adjustment into the surrounding social environment. The philosophy of day treatment programming is based on the principles of "normalization" or "social role valorization" (Wolfensberger, 1972, 1974). These principles support the development and maintenance of skills that eventually enable retarded individuals to function independently in a community setting. Such skills would include prerequisite cognitive, physical, social, attitudinal, behavioral, and communicative skills necessary for success in the job market (Wehman, 1981). Because functional curriculum and community integration are stressed, the movement from training sites to more vocationally based programs (e.g., sheltered workshops, supported work placements, competitive employment) is a realistic goal for many retarded individuals. Day treatment programs thus combine traditional special needs curricula (e.g., activities of daily living, independent living skills, self-care, communication, and leisure skills), together with vocationally oriented training (e.g., appropriate work behaviors, travel training, and community integration), to create a clinical environment that is empowering, supportive and nonthreatening.

It is within such a context that the work of teaching actually occurs. An examination of the instructional dialogue that takes place between teaching staff and program participants is critical because it helps to illustrate how language is constructed between partners. In particular, it examines how interactions are managed, and reveals who wields the authority and power in such management. The following discussion of the uses of regulatory language in instructional settings aids in determining how positions of authority between staff and client are established. These positions, I maintain, are similar in nature to those in less-structured, more conversational interactions where, in the absence of defineable teacher–student roles, an imbalance of conversational control still prevails.

Before turning to the data on interactions between teachers and people with retardation, one must first consider the literatures on instructional discourse and conversational control.

INSTRUCTIONAL DISCOURSE

The work of several investigators interested in the "language of schooling" have provided information about instructional discourse. Duchan (1989) reviewed the literature on lessons, or discourse "events" that typically occur in classrooms. According to her review, the language of a lesson is constrained by the setting in which it occurs and so comes to possess its own set of identifying criteria. These criteria distinguish instructional discourse from more informal instructional interactions, such as free time or sharing time. Characteristics unique to instructional discourse include the following:

1. teacher-initiated directives ("OK, we can begin");
2. turn-taking routines (round robin, answering in unison, bidding for next turn, teacher nominations, teacher–student–teacher–next student);
3. teacher-controlled exchange structures (initiation–reply–evaluation); and
4. regulatory language (getting ready, keeping quiet, taking turns, doing work, staying seated).

These characteristics not only describe the types of interactions inherent to a classroom, but also provide a blueprint for obtaining and relinquishing control in an educational setting. Thus, those who impose the educational agenda must be able to determine how quickly or slowly learning occurs, and must be able to modify their teaching to encourage self-regulation in those being taught.

Blank and Milewski (1981) also identified regulatory controls that educators exercise during instruction and described a model of teacher–student discourse based on a concept of *controlled complexity*. Controlled complexity is defined as the systematic regulation of adult–child sequences in which the teacher simplifies or reformulates his or her content to reduce the extent of the mismatch between the child's conceptual resources and the actual meaning of teacher-initiated questions. These simplifying procedures are activated when the child fails to supply some specific bit of information being requested. Controlled complexity can be further described as a set of instructional principles used by teachers and internalized by children as a strategy for problem solving.

Cazden (1988) likened this type of instructional discourse to the principle of *scaffolding* (a term introduced by Bruner, 1983). In simplification sequences, the child involved in the learning process does what he or she can while the adult in the interaction works out the many details necessary to maximize learning. Studies designed to explore the role of dialogue in providing scaffolding instruction (e.g., Palinscar, 1986) suggest that teachers initially provide explanation coupled with modeling, then fade out the modeling. Teachers also promote self-evaluation and reintroduce explanation and modeling as needed (see Cazden, 1988, for a review of this literature).

This pattern of instructional interaction is fairly consistent with the notion of "institutional discourse" proposed by Agar (1985). According to Agar's model, institutional discourse is described as the nonegalitarian type of discourse that results when a member of society, operating in a *client framework*, makes contact with someone who is known to represent one of that society's recognized institutions, operating in an *institutional framework*. Although Agar's sociopolitical description of what constitutes institutional discourse is derived from courtroom and medical interview data, it is both interesting and germane to the present discussion to make comparisons to classroom discourse, given the parallels to role relationships between participants in the instructional dyad (i.e., teacher vs. student).

According to Agar, institutional discourse must accomplish three things. First, the institutional representative (i.e., teacher) "diagnoses" the client (i.e., student), in terms of a limited set of ways that the institution (i.e., school district) has for describing people, their problems, and possible solutions. Second, the institution provides "directives" (i.e., instructions) that dictate what the client must do to rectify identified problems. Finally, the institution provides a "report" (i.e., individualized educational plan—IEP), usually directed to other institutional representatives, and not necessarily in the presence of the client, which summarizes the institution's findings concerning that client.

This analysis may be viewed in light of the "ideological complex" notion proposed by Hodge and Kress (1988). These authors spoke of a "functionally related set of contradictory versions of the world, coercively imposed by one social group on another on behalf of its own distinctive interests, or subversively offered by another social group in attempts at resistance in its own interests" (p. 3).

The ideological complex can come to represent what is known as the "social order," a view of the world that simultaneously serves the interests of both dominant and subordinate groups in an interaction. Thus, both Hodge and Kress (1988) and Agar (1985) viewed control as a nonnegotiable entity between institutional classes in the social order. In contrast, the instructional models cited previously view control as a mutually attributed entity that begins in the hands of one, and that over time gets delegated into the hands of many (Blank & Milewski, 1981; Cazden 1988; Palinscar, 1986).

CONVERSATIONAL CONTROL

From outside the domain of instructional discourse, studies of the functionality of retarded speakers' interactions in non-classroom settings (Kernan & Sabsay, 1984, 1987) have demonstrated that persons with retardation exhibit limitations similar to nonretarded students in terms of conversational self-regulation. Retarded adults have been reported at times to demonstrate referencing problems by the uses of "he" or "she" on first mention in a conversation (Kernan & Sabsay,

1987). They have likewise been reported to supply inadequate background information when giving directions to nonretarded persons (Kernan & Sabsay, 1984). Given the communicative breakdowns that result, retarded adults come to rely on the ability of other (nonretarded) speakers to regulate the conversation and/or to do the repair work needed. Just as teachers assume a more active role in regulating an instructional interaction to maximize learning, so too do nonretarded speakers take a more facilitative role in seeking clarification at times of confusion to better understand the pragmatic intention of retarded speaker utterances in non-classroom interactions.

Sabsay and Kernan (1983) referred to this phenomenon as a breakdown in "communicative design," or the failure on the part of the retarded speakers to at times take into account the informational needs of their listeners across linguistic, social, and interpersonal settings. In so doing, retarded speakers fail to utilize the rules of speaking that apply in given speaking situations and thus come to rely on "external guidance" in the retrieving of requisite cognitive information necessary for effectively performing communicative tasks. This view is consistent with the description just provided of teachers regulating and controlling instructional interactions. It acknowledges the role of nonretarded speakers in more conversational dyads to control the interaction in order to avoid possible misunderstandings.

In a study by Bedrosian and Prutting (1978) that looked specifically at the issue of control in several nonretarded–retarded speaker dyads, different aspects of control were investigated. In that investigation, the authors sought to define *dominance* or *submissiveness* in an exchange by looking at the communicative interactions of four adults with moderate-to-severe mental retardation across four conversational settings: with a speech-language pathologist (SLP), with parents, with peers, and with a normally intelligent but younger aged child. Results of that study concluded that adults with mental retardation could express control in four different ways:

1. having the majority of their dominant or submissive bids for action accepted by the respondent,
2. not allowing a listener to respond to a bid,
3. using "chaining" (repeated question-asking), and
4. using "arching" (answering questions with questions).

Bedrosian and Prutting determined that retarded subjects were capable of expressing control via the same types of self-regulatory routines as nonretarded speakers, although to a lesser degree. Relevant to my present study, the types of control exhibited by each retarded subject in the Bedrosian and Prutting work varied as a function of the particular setting (i.e., the partner with whom they were conversationally engaged). One subject expressed control by having the majority of his bids accepted in parental and child interactions. Another subject exhibited this type of control (bid acceptance) with all interlocutors except his peers, whereas a third subject displayed this control mechanism with all participants but her mother. The final subject displayed control via bid acceptance in every interaction.

The second type of control, not allowing the listener to respond to a bid, was exhibited by one retarded subject with all participants but the SLP; and by a different subject while interacting with his SLP, parents, and peers. Another subject expressed this control mechanism in interactions with her mother, whereas the final subject, again, was able to exercise this control type with all participants.

All but one of the subjects expressed control via arching: one subject with the SLP; one with his parents and child; and one with her peers and child. Only one subject did not express control via chaining, while the remaining subjects used chaining in two interactions each: Two subjects used chaining with their parents and the child; and one used chaining with her peers and the child.

As useful as the Bedrosian and Prutting (1978) study is in determining conversational settings in which retarded individuals are able to exercise control, it fails to take into account the instructional setting as a valid location in which to conduct similar observations. The present investigation was thus undertaken to focus further on the issues of control and intention in instructional discourse with the adult retarded population.

In order to address the issues of self-regulatory abilities and interactional control of adult retarded speakers, a descriptive-analytic study was conducted at an adult day treatment program for mildly to moderately retarded individuals. Videotape procedures were employed to capture two different levels of instructional interactions involving program participants and their nonretarded instructors.

RESEARCH METHODS

Subjects

Ten adults (5 male and 5 female) with diagnoses in the range of mild-to-moderate mental retardation, as determined by performance on psychological test assessments and adaptive behavior composite scores, were selected to participate in the present study. Subject selection was further determined on the basis of the following:

1. sensory capability: no identifiable problems with hearing or vision, as indicated in case records;
2. verbal ability: unimpaired intelligibility at the level of conversational speech, based on Shriberg and Kwiatkowski's (1982) phonological criteria;
3. native language: English;

4. age: chronological age between 21;0 and 50;0 years; and
5. passable performance on functional language assessment tool (Let's Talk Inventory; Wiig, 1982).

Male and female instructors were included in the study based on their willingness to participate in videotaping procedures. Instructional staff were classified at either the senior instructional or instructional level, which reflected both proven competence in teaching, as well as longevity with the host agency. Each instructor in the study possessed a baccalaureate degree.

Design

A repeated measures procedure was incorporated in the study. Subjects were pseudo-randomly assigned to instructors, based on subject availability on the days of taping. The subjects with mental retardation were engaged in two separate teaching conditions: *lessons* and *joint problem-solving* sessions.

Under the formal lesson condition, two instructors, one male and one female, were selected to work with five subjects each from the total subject population. The female instructor taught Game 1, whereas the male taught Game 2 to respective subjects.

Under the joint problem-solving condition, half the subjects engaged in one informal craft activity (1), whereas the other half engaged in a different craft activity (2). Ten different instructors were employed under this condition, and paired with each of the 10 subjects. This was done to guarantee that neither party in the dyad held any advantage over the other in terms of possessing prior knowledge about the activity.

The teachers in the study are displayed in Table 7.1 as "T," and the retarded clients are displayed as "C." The numbers used under the lesson condition indicate the actual pairs: The first teacher (T1) is paired with each of the 5 clients (C1 to C5), whereas the second teacher (T2) is paired with each of the remaining clients (C6 to C10). Under the problem-solving condition, each of the numbers (1–10) next to the "T" indicate the 10 different teachers used across two craft activities. Similarly, the numbers (1–10) next to the "C" indicate the 10 different clients across the two craft activities. T1 was matched with C1; T2 with C2; and so on.

Instructional Cells

Formal lessons were selected on the basis of their being representative "events" in the daily routine of the day treatment setting. Each event possessed its own set of identifying criteria (Duchan, 1989), that served to distinguish it from patterns that existed in less formal classroom interactions, such as morning check-in or break-time. Joint problem-solving interactions, on the other hand, were more conversational in nature. Neither of the dyad members involved in a joint problem-solving

TABLE 7.1
Research Design

Lesson				Problem Solving	
Game 1		*Game 2*		*Craft 1*	*Craft 2*
	C1		C6		
	C2		C7	T: 1 2 3 4 5	6 7 8 9 10
T1	C3	T2	C8		
	C4		C9	C: 1 2 3 4 5	6 7 8 9 10
	C5		C10		

Note. T = teacher; C = client

task possessed prior information about the task, thereby making them less likely to know the "right" way to approach the problem to be solved.

1. Formal Lesson Game 1: One instructor was directed to teach her five participating subjects the card game "Old Maid."
2. Formal Lesson Game 2: The second instructor was directed to teach his game of "Super Tic Tac Toe."

These games were selected because subjects were familiar with card and board games that were included in their recreational therapy curriculum. Pilot investigations (Domingo, 1991) have suggested that card and board games were a source of enjoyment for program participants. They were thus considered conducive to eliciting the control bids of interest.

3. Joint Problem-Solving Activity 1: Prior to the arrival of the five different subject–teacher dyads, two boxes were set up at the work area, each containing half the materials needed to complete a "terrarium planter."
4. Joint Problem-Solving Activity 2: Two additional boxes were set up in the work area prior to the arrival of the remaining subject–teacher dyads, each containing half the materials needed to complete a craft "embroidery hoop."

For each activity, an already completed object (terrarium or hoop), was placed in plain sight of the participants as a working model. Each of the dyads was given the general instruction to complete another one like the one they saw. They were told to work together and share materials as needed.

Verbal Bids of Control

The occurrence and distribution of verbal "summonses," as initially described by Bedrosian and Prutting (1978) and further modified for the present study, were evaluated to determine the degree of control that either retarded or nonretarded speakers demonstrated in different instructional interactions. Such verbal summonses included dominant and submissive bids.

Dominant Bids

Strong Directives (SD). SDs are initiatory utterances that compel or request the listener to carry out some action, for example,

Put your name on that one// (SD)

Just draw a circle// (SD)

Weak Directives (WD). WDs are responsive utterances produced in conjunction with strong directives that, in turn, compel the listener to carry out some activity; contextualized utterances produced in the carrying out of the activity that ensure the continuation of the activity; or utterances that reflect some curricular or activity-specific meaning, for example,

Tell me what you want// (SD) *or* Have any 3's?//

Give me the green one// (WD)   Go Fish// (WD)

or I deal the cards// (WD)

We can put it in the cup// (WD)

Submissive Bids

Uninformed Questions (UQ). UQs are utterances that request needed information and that are dependent on the respondent for supplying it; or utterances that request opinions, for example,

What do we need to start this job?// (UQ)

How do you think it's coming out?// (UQ)

Interrater Reliability

Following transcription and coding procedures of the database, 10% of the transcribed data were coded for their dominant and submissive control bids by an independent rater who had a master's degree in clinical psychology and 3 year's experience in working with an adult developmentally disabled/mentally retarded population. This rater was given 2 hours of instruction by the study's investigator and could use videotapes to assist in her coding of transcribed utterances. Interrater reliability of 92% (agreement regarding the coding of utterances) was attained.

RESULTS AND DISCUSSION

In the discourse analysis that follows, both quantitative and qualitative measurements are reported. Statistical findings examining the adult retarded speakers' abilities across instructional contexts are not presented. Rather, the findings examining the content of retarded speaker utterances with respect to the *pragmatic intentions* of their utterances are discussed. In comparison to the nonretarded speakers, retarded speakers were significantly less able to establish conversational control. Interestingly, retarded speakers were able to express the same types of dominant and submissive bids as their nonretarded counterparts, although to a lesser degree. Use of qualitative measures was advantageous in that it revealed a certain depth and complexity to the retarded speakers' utterances in the informal instructional context. Moreover, these utterances were considered as sophisticated as those of nonretarded speakers in expressing pragmatic intention.

Quantitative Measures

All turns produced in the 20 observational sessions across instructional conditions were transcribed and segmented into utterances, following Loban's (1976) criteria of what constitutes a "communication unit" (C-unit; each is an independent clause with all its modifiers). Following that, utterances were coded according to dominant or submissive bid criteria, and the means and standard deviations for dependent variables of control (SD, WD, UQ) were tabulated (see Table 7.2).

Following the coding of data into dominant and submissive bids, separate analyses of variance (ANOVAs) were conducted to compare results obtained in the different teaching conditions (see Table 7.3).

Teachers working with persons with retardation produced significantly more weak directives, a dominant bid type, during formal lessons than during joint

TABLE 7.2
Summary of Bid-Type by Instructional Condition

	Lessons		*Joint Problem Solving*	
Variables	*M*	*(SD)*	*M*	*(SD)*
SD (T)	18.9	(10.9)	23.0	(13.9)
WD (T)	55.0	(9.8)	34.5	(20.1)
UQ (T)	5.1	(3.6)	13.9	(7.5)
SD (C)	1.2	(1.03)	4.5	(5.3)
WD (C)	9.9	(6.7)	16.2	(14.9)
UQ (C)	3.7	(4.2)	7.9	(9.3)

Note. T = teacher; C = client; SD = strong directives; WD = weak directives; UQ = uninformed questions; *M* = mean; *SD* = standard deviations.

TABLE 7.3
ANOVA Contrasts Across Conditions

Variables	*Degrees of Freedom*	*Lesson × Problem Solving*
SD (T)	*F* (1,17)	1.15
WD (T)	*F* (1,17)	13.36**
UQ (T)	*F* (1,17)	3.79~
SD (C)	*F* (1,17)	0.20
WD (C)	*F* (1,17)	0.001***
UQ (C)	*F* (1,17)	0.15

~$p < .10$ (trend); *$p < .05$; **$p < .01$; ***$p < .001$.

Note. T = teacher; C = client; SD = strong directives; WD = weak directives; UQ = uninformed questions.

problem solving [$F(1, 17) = 13.36, p < .01$]. However, teachers tended to produce more uninformed questions, a submissive control bid, during the informal setting than during formal game instructions [$F(1, 17) = 3.79$, $p < .10$]. Subjects with retardation in either condition did not exhibit significant findings with respect to control bids produced, although they showed consistency in increasing their dominant and submissive bids as they moved from the formal to the informal instructional situation with their nonretarded counterparts (see Table 7.2 for a comparison of means across conditions).

For the teachers involved, these findings were predictable, given that in formal lessons a more straightforward and directorial style of instruction is expected. By contrast, the absence of a formal agenda in joint problem solving resulted in a higher number of submissive bids by teachers. These results reflect the greater informality and collegiality of the informal interaction.

The subjects with retardation in the study showed no significant differences in the expression of either dominant or submissive bids for control. However, they were still able to produce the same types of control bids as their nonretarded counterparts, though to a lesser degree. A qualitative examination of their utterances revealed how the informal lesson context fostered the use of certain intentionality forms in the retarded speakers' expression of control bids.

Qualitative Analysis

The following section describes the dominant and submissive bids produced by the subjects with retardation and their instructors. Such an analysis of pragmatic intentions provides insight into what the different participants are capable of accomplishing in their interpersonal interactions.

Strong Directives (SD). Across the formal and informal lessons conducted, the subjects with retardation and their nonretarded counterparts expressed dominant bids in the form of SDs. That teachers should produce such bids is not surprising. (One could generally assume that teachers possess, at the very least, some practice with giving directions.) That the speakers with retardation were also able to express certain SD forms was of interest.

Whenever teachers expressed SDs during formal lessons, their intention was to initiate some instructional sequence, either to provide instruction or to direct attention to some presented task, examples of what Cazden (1988) called "curricular language." When individuals with mental retardation expressed an SD in the formal lesson context, they did so either to regulate the direction and flow of information or, in some cases, to request repetition of the task being carried out. Therefore, the intentionality underlying the production of their bids in formal lessons was qualitatively different from the intentionality forms expressed by the teachers. However, during joint problem solving, the expression of SDs by the subjects with retardation (C) reflected the same intentionality forms (instructing; directing attention) as those expressed by the teachers (T) conducting formal lessons. Some examples follow:

1. *Teacher-Produced SD Bid/Lesson (initiatory)*
   T: *Look at the board carefully* // (SD)
   Cause you don't want me to win // right? /
   C: No //
   T: Why don't you show me // *Take some* // (SD)
   and show me the different ways you can win // (SD)
2. *Client-Produced SD Bid/Lesson (regulatory)*
   C: *You'll have to explain this slowly to me* // (SD)
   So I know what I'm doing //
   T: OK / you got one step is to take out the Queens //
3. *Client-Produced SD Bid/Problem Solve (initiatory)*
   T: Unscrew this a little bit //
   C: *You have to put this one in first* // (SD)
   Put that right here // (SD)
   T: OK/ let's take a look //
   C: You have to uh / What are you doing? //
   You have to . *wait a minute* // (SD)
   You have to put that underneath // (SD)

As these examples show, persons with retardation used dominant SD bids not only to regulate the direction and flow of instruction to aid in comprehension (Example 2, from the formal lesson), but also used SDs to provide instruction to nonretarded partners (Example 3, from joint problem solving). As such, the latter example demonstrates the capacity of the subject with retardation to initiate instructional sequences and to control the interaction rather than merely serve a regulatory role, a skill not exhibited during formal lessons. Thus, informal settings may be more conducive to eliciting the same types of SD bids in retarded subjects as in teachers.

Weak Directives (WD). In the formal lesson, subjects with retardation produced dominant WD bids that were explicit in nature (i.e., WD bids that consisted of direct statements produced in response to teacher-initiated strong directives, as per the definition of the bid type). Such WDs during formal lessons did not consist of either indirect statements or question forms that suggested compliance. Some examples of teacher and subject explicit WD bids follow:

1. *Teacher-Produced WD Bid/Lesson (explicit form)*
   C: So let's try it again // (SD)
   T: *OK/ we'll play one more game //* (WD)
2. *Client-Produced WD Bid/Lesson (explicit form)*
   T: Where should you put your piece now? //
   C: *Put it over there //* (WD)

In contrast to these explicit WD bids, implicit WDs were viewed as being more suggestive in nature, serving to elicit the same desired responses as explicit WD bid types, but more indirectly. Qualitative differences in how the two groups of speakers were able to express control with WD bids during formal lessons were evident. The differences between speaker groups disappeared in the informal, more egalitarian interaction, however.

Implicit forms of WD bids that signaled control for their users included: suggestive questions, orienting questions, and modal verbs. Although the subjects with retardation in formal lessons did not exhibit these variations of the WD bid, they were observed employing them in the joint problem-solving context. Some examples that show how suggested actions are taken up through less direct means follow:

3. *Teacher-Produced WD Bid/Lesson (implicit : question)*
   T: If you get one in each of the corners /
   C: Yeah? //
   T: *Wanna put that one in there? //* (WD)
   C: OK // (client places piece)
   T: You can win //
4. *Client-Produced WD Bid/Problem Solve (implicit: question)*
   T: See where we have to cut about //
   C: [How about right over] *How about right here? //* (WD)
   T: Right about there? //
   C: There //

5. *Teacher-Produced WD Bid/Lesson (implicit : orienting)*
   T: OK / *do you notice something though?* // (WD)
   [look at my] [before you make that move]
   You sure you want to make that move? // (WD)
   C: yeah //
   T: Look / if you make that move /
   Know what I'm doing? // (WD)
   I'm gonna put mine here// and I'll win //
6. *Client-Produced WD Bid/Problem Solve (implicit: orienting)*
   T: OK / This is what we're gonna do //
   This is what we go by //
   C: *Now know what I have to do?* // (WD)
   I'll hafta put it in a frame //

Such examples from the data cannot be identified as either fact-finding or request-for-information type questions (Examples 3 and 4). Other questions (Examples 5 and 6) appear to serve an orienting function (where the speaker producing the utterance seeks to re-direct attention to some given task or aspect of the activity). As a result, they are considered task-related in nature. This implies that some action or activity be carried out by the listener to ensure continuation of the task itself. Posed as questions or requests for action, these utterances aid the listener in focusing in on some aspect of the game or activity that might have been missed. As such, they are considered WD forms.

Finally, other implicit WD bids, manifested in the form of modal verbs, also imply that actions should be taken. The modals "would," "could," or "should," when used in the context of "how a move ought to be carried out," make an appeal to the listener to follow through with some indicated action. For example:

7. *Teacher-Produced WD Bid/Lesson (implicit : modal)*
   T: *You should look at what I'm trying to do* // (WD)
   C: Yeah //
   T: *I would put that here to block me* // (WD)
   C: Yeah // (places piece on mat board)
   T: If you look over here / *You could get four in a row* // (WD)
8. *Client-Produced WD Bid/Problem Solve (implicit : modal)*
   T: OK / you pick which horse you wanna use //
   C: *That could be good* // (WD)
   This could be good // (WD)

What these examples from the informal setting suggest is that speakers with retardation are able to employ a wider range of communicative behaviors and intention forms in comparison to their performance in formal lessons. The demonstrated ability of these retarded speakers to exhibit both explicit and implicit WD forms during informal teaching that are qualitatively similar to the intentionality forms expressed by teachers may be a reflection of the more egalitarian setting in which the interaction occurs. The informal instructional setting would thus be recommended for optimally facilitating expressions of pragmatic intentions and communicative competence.

Uninformed Questions (UQ). Instructors used UQs, a submissive form of control, sparingly during formal lessons, but demonstrated a trend increase in their use as the setting became more egalitarian. Their UQ bids during lessons frequently were located at the beginnings of sessions to determine whether subjects possessed knowledge of the games about to be presented. Interestingly, the retarded subjects did not employ similar initializing sequences at the start of the interaction to determine nonretarded speakers' knowledge concerning either a game in the formal lesson context, or an activity in the problem-solving context. They did, however, employ UQ bids at points other than at the beginnings of sessions, to solicit missing information from their nonretarded counterparts. For example:

1. *Teacher-Produced UQ Bid/Lesson (initializing sequence)*
   T: This is Super Tic Tac Toe //
   You ever play regular Tic Tac Toe? // (UQ)
   C: Yeah / I've done that //
2. *Teacher-Produced UQ Bid/Problem Solve (missing info)*
   T: *OK / So what do you think we have to do? //* (UQ)
   C: I don't know //
   T: *What is underneath that material? //* (UQ)
   C: More material //
   T: *There's nothing left in your box? //* (UQ)
3. *Client-Produced UQ Bid/Lesson (missing info)*
   T: These pairs can tell us who is gonna win the game //
   C: *So I hafta do the same? //* (UQ)
   T: uh huh // I have two kings //
   I don't wanna look at your hand to help you //
   C: *Well / do I put down [the same] spades too? //* (UQ)
   T: Whatever you have two of //
4. *Client-Produced UQ Bid/Problem Solve (missing info)*
   T: What's on top of this? //
   What kind of thing? //
   C: *Glass? //* (UQ)
   T: No / there's no glass // Take a look at it //
   What's on top of here // What's around it? //
   C: *What is this called? //* (UQ)
   T: I don't know //

Still other applications of submissive control bids expressed via UQ types by teachers and retarded subjects came in the form of requesting opinions (nontask-related talking) regarding either a separate activity, or the well-being of listeners themselves. In the examples of teachers asking subjects "what they thought" about something outside the testing area, or "how they were," instructors departed from a routine they had established during formal instruction, where they engaged only minimally in nontask-related talk. Indeed, teachers only engaged in such a manner when induced to do so by subjects seeking personal attention (Example 5), but refrained from it by-and-large during the formal lesson context. Retarded subjects likewise used nontask-related UQ bids infrequently during formal lessons (Example 7), but made greater use of this question type during the joint problem-solving sessions. The data thus suggest that both speaker groups were sensitive to the formality of the lesson setting, given the infrequent occurrence of such nontask-related question forms under that condition. These utterances, usually concerned either with the location or well-being of another person from the day treatment program, constituted a submissive form of control in that they compelled the listener to quit the activity temporarily in order to respond. Some examples follow:

5. *Teacher-Produced UQ Bid/Lesson (nontask-related talk)*
   C: Where is Jim? //
   T: Up in the AP Room //
   C: Is he gonna be here Monday too? //
   T: Sure// *Are you gonna be here Monday?* // (UQ)
   C: Yeah // When is your vacation Lisa? //
   T: August 14 // *When is your vacation?* // (UQ)
   C: uh . . . . I don't know //
6. *Teacher-Produced UQ Bid/Problem Solve (nontask-related talk)*
   T: Yeah / the Gap program has lots of Rec activities //
   C: yup //
   T: *You do dancing and things like that there?* // (UQ)
   C: Yup / and I do that very good //
7) *Client-Produced UQ Bid/Lesson (nontask-related talk)*
   T: Let's try a card game now // OK? /
   C: uh huh // *Who's working in your classroom?* // (UQ)
   T: Jim //
   C: *Where is Jim?* // (UQ)
8. *Client-Produced UQ Bid/Problem Solve (nontask-related talk)*
   T: OK / so cut it carefully //
   C: *Victor coming in today?* // (UQ)
   T: No / Victor is on vacation //
   C: *How long does he have?* // (UQ)
   T: He's got one more week //

CONCLUSIONS AND CLINICAL IMPLICATIONS

The present investigation examined the ability of adults with mental retardation to exercise control in instructional interactions. It may be posited that certain limitations inherent to an instructional paradigm make it difficult to capture more naturalistic discourse between adults with mental retardation and their day treatment instructors, thus biasing one's view of the interactive style of the individuals studied. However, as stated earlier, I suggest that the verbal interactions occurring in the instructional settings under investigation may parallel conversational interactions one finds in the absence of defineable "teacher–student" roles, where an imbalance of control between speaker groups prevails. Thus, instructional interactions may be as good a barometer as any to provide insights into the self-regulatory ability of adults with mental retardation to gain control in an interaction.

Statistically, adults with mental retardation did not exercise interactional control over nonretarded interlocutors in either of the formal or informal instructional settings. In comparison, teachers were observed displaying more dominant bids for control in the formal interaction and more submissive bids in the interaction as the informality of the setting increased. Thus, limiting the investigation to a quantitative analysis might lead one to conclude that speakers with retardation are deficient in their ability to exercise control in instructional settings. In addition, it might also suggest that retarded speakers are subject to the influences of other (nonretarded) speakers in the interaction to aid in the retrieval of necessary cognitive strategies needed to display appropriate communicative design (Sabsay & Kernan, 1983).

Although it is not always clear why mentally retarded speakers rely more heavily at times on other people to regulate a conversational interaction for them, Sabsay and Kernan (1983) pointed out the general ease with which an interaction can be taken over and controlled by the conversation's nonretarded participant. They cited several studies (Buium, Rynders, & Turnure, 1974; Marshall, Hegrenes, & Goldstein, 1973; Sabsay, 1979) that demonstrated how nonretarded speakers directed and controlled conversations with either unrelated adults with Down syndrome or with offspring who were mentally retarded. Sabsay and Kernan stated the following:

> It is easy to imagine a lifetime of linguistic experience in which a retarded individual has had most of the verbal interactions he has engaged in controlled and directed by others. It should not be surprising that the result of such experience would be the failure to develop the ability to self-regulate, and a reliance on the regulation of others. (p. 293)

The qualitative analysis, by contrast, revealed that retarded persons were able to express dominant and submissive bids for action and attention that were similar to the types of bids produced by teachers. This became most evident when an examination of their utterances' pragmatic intentions in informal instructional interactions were explored.

In particular, the subjects with retardation changed in their expression of strong directives from one interaction to the next, using utterances that initiated and facilitated the activity and that did not simply mark or regulate it in some passive manner. How weak directives were expressed changed as well, from being explicit or straightforward in nature, to being implicit or suggestive in getting the listener to carry out some action. Finally, with respect to uninformed questions, it was noted that the subjects with retardation increased their use of nontask-related talking that reflected something of the collegiality and egalitarianism of the informal lesson context.

From such an analysis of the pragmatic intentions of speaker utterances, it was shown how adults with retardation possessed an underlying potential for exercising control in instructional interactions. Their utterances signaling control were qualitatively similar to the linguistic control markers used by nonretarded speakers. Across both instructional conditions, the subjects with retardation were seen producing a range of regulatory/initiatory strong directives, explicit/implicit weak directives, and task/nontask-related uninformed questions that teachers were likewise credited with producing. The more informal the setting, the more likely it appeared that subjects with retardation would become facilitative in their interactional styles. Such observations would recommend the informal interaction in eliciting different utterance types that span a wide range of pragmatic intentions.

Armed with the preceding observations, and aware of the scientific findings concerning the communicative capabilities of the adult developmentally disabled/mentally retarded population, the task now becomes one of utilizing the knowledge gained to further enhance the discourse skills of such a group. Edgerton (1967) may have been correct in asserting that adults with mental retardation have a disposition for learned helplessness where, as a result of their inherent "lower standing" in the community, such individuals are further made to develop into dependent and unquestioning members of the society. If this is true, then responsibility must begin to shift to those in more authoritative positions (i.e., teachers or clinicians) to create situations that empower retarded individuals to make choices for themselves.

The key may lie in the interactional setting. As this study demonstrates, formal instructional interactions fall short in being able to provide opportunities to retarded individuals to exert control in situations where "others" (teachers) occupy the position of authority. As such, the typical "events" that occur in a classroom, as detailed by Duchan (1989), may not be the most effective means of training discourse skills. Because informality in a setting appears conducive to eliciting a range of pragmatic intentions in retarded speaker utterances, more time needs to be spent in developing informal dialogue skills.

During classroom interactions, teachers and clinicians may set up various scenarios that expose the retarded participants to more creative teaching alternatives. Such alternatives may include role playing (where participants enact mock situations of people meeting and interacting under various conditions); problem solving (where participants report on what they would do in different situations to avoid conflict); and/or modeling (where participants demonstrate for one another both correct and incorrect ways of expressing themselves in real-life situations). In addition, whenever possible, persons with retardation should be provided with opportunities within the community (at restaurants, on the bus, at shopping malls) to practice discourse abilities learned through informal, creative means. This would go a long way toward achieving the carryover that clinicians value but find difficult to induce in therapeutic interactions.

The important work of training discourse skills in the adult retarded speaker lies ahead. Instructional interactions as presently exist in day treatment programs (that are highly regulated and monitored by other, nonretarded persons in authority) should be re-evaluated and revised. Only when more empowering opportunities are made available to retarded individuals for making habilitative choices can one expect significant changes to occur in their independent level of functioning. In the absence of such opportunities, persons with mental retardation will forever remain compromised and dependent citizens of the society.

REFERENCES

Agar, M. (1985). Institutional discourse. *Text, 5,* 147–168.

Anderson-Levitt, K., & Platt, M. (1984). *The speech of mentally retarded adults in contrastive settings* (Working Paper # 28). Los Angeles: Socio-Behavioral Group, M tal Retardation Research Center, UCLA.

Bedrosian, J. (1988). Adults who are mildly tc moderately mentally retarded: Communicative performance, assessment and intervention. In S. Calculator & J. Bedrosian (Eds.), *Communication assessment and intervention for adults with mental retardation* (pp. 265–307). Boston: College-Hill Press.

Bedrosian, J., & Prutting, C. (1978). Communicative performance of mentally retarded adults in four conversational settings. *Journal of Speech and Hearing Research, 21,* 79–95.

Blank, M., & Milewski, J. (1981). Applying psycholinguistic concepts to the treatment of an autistic child. *Applied Psycholinguistics, 2,* 65–84.

Blount, W. (1968). Language and the more severely retarded: A review. *American Journal of Mental Deficiency, 1,* 21–29.

Bruner, J. (1983). *Child's talk: Learning to use language.* New York: Norton.

Buium, N., Rynders, J., & Turnure, J. (1974). Early maternal linguistic environment of normal and Down's Syndrome language-learning children. *American Journal of Mental Deficiency, 79,* 52–58.

Cazden, C. (1988). *Classroom discourse: The language of teaching & learning.* Portsmouth, NH: Heinemann Educational Books.

Domingo, R. (1991). *The influence of setting and interlocutor on the ability of adult retarded speakers to exhibit control in an instructional context.* Unpublished doctoral dissertation, The City University of New York, Graduate Center, New York.

Duchan, J. (1989). *Discourse and the classroom*. Short course presented at the 29th annual convention of the New York State Speech-Language-Hearing Association, Kiamesha Lake, NY.

Edgerton, R. (1967). *The cloak of competence: Stigma in the lives of the retarded*. Berkeley: University of California Press.

Graffam, J. (1983). *About ostriches coming out of Communist China: Meanings, functions and frequencies of typical interactions in group meetings*. (Working Paper #27). Los Angeles: Socio-Behavioral Group, Mental Retardation Research Center, UCLA.

Hodge, R., & Kress, G. (1988). *Social semiotics*. Ithaca, NY: Cornell University Press.

Kernan, K., & Sabsay, S. (1982). Semantic deficiencies in the narratives of mildly retarded speakers. *Semiotica, 42*, 169–193.

Kernan, K., & Sabsay, S. (1984). Getting there: Directions given by mildly retarded and nonretarded adults. In R. Edgerton (Ed.), *Lives in process: Mildly retarded adults in a large city*. Washington DC: AAMD Monograph No. 6.

Kernan, K., & Sabsay, S. (1987). Referential first mention in narratives by mildly retarded adults. *Research in Developmental Disabilities, 8*, 361–370.

Linder, S. (1978a). Language context and the evaluation of the verbal competence of mentally retarded (Working Paper # 1). Los Angeles: Socio-Behavioral Group, Mental Retardation Research Center, UCLA.

Linder, S. (1978b). The perception and management of "trouble" in "normal-retardate" conversations (Working Paper # 5). Los Angeles: Socio-Behavioral Group, Mental Retardation Research Center, UCLA.

Loban, W. (1976). *Language development: Kindergarten through grade 12* (Res. Rep. No. 18). Urbana, IL: National Council of Teachers of English.

Marshall, N., Hegrenes, J., & Goldstein, S. (1973). Verbal interactions: Mothers & their nonretarded children. *American Journal of Mental Deficiency, 77*, 415–419.

Palinscar, A. (1986). The role of dialogue in providing scaffold instruction. *Educational Psychologist, 21*, 73–98.

Platt, M. (1984). *Displaying competence: Peer interaction in a group home for retarded adults*. (Working Paper # 29). Los Angeles: Socio-Behavioral Group, Mental Retardation Research Center, UCLA.

Sabsay, S. (1979). *Communicative competence in Down's Syndrome adults*. Unpublished doctoral dissertation, University of California, Los Angeles.

Sabsay, S., & Kernan, K. (1983). Communicative design in the speech of mildly retarded adults. In K. Kernan, M. Begab, & R. Edgerton (Eds.), *Environments and behavior: The adaptation of mentally retarded persons* (pp. 283–294). Baltimore, MD: University Park Press.

Schegloff, E., Jefferson, G., & Sacks, H. (1977). The preference for self-correction in the organization of repair in conversation. *Language, 53*, 361–382.

Schiefelbusch, R. (Ed.). (1972). *Language of the mentally retarded*. Baltimore, MD: University Park Press.

Shriberg, L., & Kwiatkowski, J (1982). Phonological disorders III: A procedure for assessing severity of involvement. *Journal of Speech & Hearing Disorders, 47*, 256–270.

Turner, J. (1982). *Workshop society: Ethnographic observations in a work setting for retarded adults*. (Working Paper # 20). Los Angeles: Socio-Behavioral Group, Mental Retardation Research Center, UCLA.

Wehman, P. (1981). *Competitive employment: New horizons for severely disabled individuals*. Baltimore, MD: Paul H. Brookes.

Wiig, E. (1982). *Let's talk inventory for adolescents*. Columbus, OH: Charles E. Merrill.

Wolfensberger, W. (1972). *The principle of normalization in human services*. Toronto: National Institute on Mental Retardation.

Wolfensberger, W. (1974). Social role valorization: A proposed new term for the principle of normalization. *Mental Retardation, 21*, 234–239.

Chapter 8

Oral Story Production in Adults With Learning Disabilities

Froma P. Roth
University of Maryland

Nancy J. Spekman
Marianne Frostig Center for Educational Therapy
Paseadena, CA

Studies of young adults with learning disabilities consistently reveal large high school drop out rates (Cronin & Patton, in press; Zigmond & Thornton, 1985), repeated unsuccessful attempts at college and training programs, unemployment, employment in low status jobs, and financial dependence (Haring, Lovett, & Smith, 1990; Patton & Palloway, 1992; Spekman, Goldberg, & Herman, 1992). These findings make it increasingly clear that learning disabilities are not outgrown and do not disappear with age, even with consistent intervention. Thus, it is not surprising that there is a growing body of evidence that many of the problems experienced by children with learning disabilities are chronic and persist into adolescence and adulthood. Proliferating research findings show ongoing difficulties in numerous areas including social and emotional status, cognition, academics, and oral language.

Specific deficits have been identified in the areas of self-concept, self-esteem, and social acceptance and adjustment (Buchanan & Wolf, 1986; Chesler, 1982; Hoffman et al., 1987; La Greca, 1987; Silver, 1984; Vaughn & La Greca, 1988). In addition, attentional deficits and problems in conceptual thinking and problem solving have been shown to be continuing problems for adults with learning disabilities. Adult outcome studies also have documented lasting academic problems in word recognition and reading comprehension (Johnson, 1987a), written composition (Johnson, 1987b), and mathematical operations and applications (Blalock, 1987; Rogan & Hartman, 1990). Finally, problems with oral language are chronic among learning disabled (LD) adults. Among the most well-documented difficulties are syntactic errors, reduced syntactic complexity

(Johnson, 1982), and difficulties with the organization and formulation of sentences and oral text (Blalock, 1982, 1987).

Although many of the problems that have been observed in the adult LD population are in the same domains as those demonstrated by school-age children and adolescents with learning disabilities, the precise nature and characteristics of the difficulties may change over time. For example, it has been noted that oral language continues to cause problems for individuals with learning disabilities across the life span; however, the exact nature of these problems has not been studied in a systematic manner.

The area of focus in this chapter is on narrative discourse, a particular aspect of oral language. Narrative discourse is a major form of human communication and refers to extended units of spoken or written language. It includes such forms as stories, descriptions, explanations, and exposition. To construct narratives, an individual must have a rule system and framework for generating the narrative form and strategies for adjusting and accommodating to different listeners and audiences.

The most widely studied form of narration is the story. Research studies that have focused on the story form indicate that LD children have a variety of problems with narrative processing, including story memory or recall (Crais & Chapman, 1987; Graybeal, 1981), literal and inferential story comprehension (Hansen, 1978; Oakhill, 1984), and story production (Merritt, & Liles, 1987; Roth & Spekman, 1986; Westby, 1982). Empirical information regarding the narrative discourse skills of adults with learning disabilities is scant. The data that are available come primarily from studies that have focused on the gist recall abilities of college students. In general, the results indicate that the LD college samples, like younger LD subjects, preserve the order of events in a story with the same degree of accuracy and exhibit the same pattern of story organization as their normally achieving counterparts. However, discrepant findings have been reported with respect to the amount of information recalled from a story. Worden, Malmgren, and Gabourie (1982) indicated that their LD subjects recalled significantly less information from stories than nondisabled peers. In contrast, Worden and Nakamura (1982) found overall recall to be equivalent in normally achieving and LD subject groups.

Although there is no information, to date, on the nature of the story production abilities of adults with learning disabilities, it is logical to suspect that such difficulties persist into adulthood. Three main reasons underlie this suspicion. First, narration of all types is a particularly demanding discourse activity, far exceeding the demands of conversational discourse in several important ways. Successful narration requires the ability to produce extended units of text that contain an organized sequence of events and ideas that lead to a logical conclusion. Further, narratives require the manipulation of numerous pieces of information simultaneously. Specifically, with respect to storytelling, the narrator must provide information about the setting and context of a story, introduce the protagonist and any other characters, identify a conflict that precipitates the story, provide an account of the plans made and steps taken to attain the goal, and specify the outcome or resolution. Often, stories are composed of multiple subplots or episodes, resulting in stories being embedded within stories.

Narratives also carry the expectation that the speaker maintain an oral monologue and that the listener assume a relatively passive role. Monologuing requires a great deal of perspective-taking ability on the part of the speaker who must assume the viewpoint of the listener and adjust messages accordingly. Thus, the communicative responsibility in narrative discourse falls squarely of the shoulders of the speaker to generate a clear, coherent, and complete story.

The second main reason for predicting persistent story production problems in LD adults is that LD students in early adolescence (i.e., 12;0–13;11 years) have been shown to evidence significant difficulties with story production. Many of their difficulties are the same as those exhibited by considerably younger children with learning disabilities. Roth and Spekman (1986) analyzed several aspects of spontaneously generated oral stories of a sample of LD and normally achieving early adolescent youngsters. One involved a story grammar analysis of orally produced stories. A story grammar describes the internal structure of a story by specifying the components of a story and a set of rules that underlie the order and relationships among story components. Thus, the story grammar proportedly represents the knowledge of story structure possessed by individuals. Presumably, the individual utilizes this information when presented with a story and when constructing one of his or her own.

Roth and Spekman's story grammar analysis revealed several significant differences in the structure of the oral stories produced by the LD and normally achieving groups, despite the demonstration of equivalent expressive syntactic abilities (Roth & Spekman, 1989b). The stories told by the LD students were shorter and contained fewer complete episodes than those produced by the normally achieving peers. Further, within an episode, the LD subjects tended to omit important information about character, setting, motive, and actions. A typical episode contained only the introduction of a protagonist(s), an event that initiated the episode, and an indication of how the episode ended. In other words, they tended to omit the entire middle portion of an episode. The middle part of episodes provides information about a character's motivations, goals, plans, and emotional states. The absence of such information detracts from the richness of stories.

A final reason to predict the persistence of narrative deficits into adulthood is the overwhelming evidence of difficulties experienced by many LD adults. Proficiency with extended units of language is a skill required in many aspects of daily life and in many occupations. For this reason, ongoing problems with narrative discourse may account, at least in part, for many of the life adjustment difficulties exhibited by learning disabled adults, including difficulties with college, problems maintaining jobs, their sizable high school drop out rate, and problems maintaining social relationships and forming lasting friendships.

A study was therefore undertaken that would permit a preliminary examination of the outcome of narrative discourse acquisition in the adult LD population. The investigation focused on one particular narrative discourse process: oral story production. Oral story production was chosen because it is one of the most demanding narrative tasks, and one that has been shown to be difficult for children and adolescents with learning disabilities. Moreover, our previous work has shown age-related changes in narrative performance in both LD and normally achieving youngsters across three age ranges. This work thus provides a baseline of performance against which to compare adult narrative performance.

The study was specifically designed to compare the oral story production abilities of adults with and without a history of learning disabilities. As part of this project, an attempt was made to assess the impact of task structure on story production through the use of two elicitation conditions: a spontaneous story production task and a story production to picture task.

METHOD

Subjects

The participants in this study were 23 adults between the ages of 30 and 50 years. One subject of an initial pool of 24 was eliminated from the study because of the nature of the story told. Twelve were adults with a history of learning disabilities (*M* = 37.8 years, *SD* = 6.2) and 11 had no history of learning disability (N-LD; *M* age = 38.5 years, *SD* = 5.8). There was a nearly equivalent proportion of males to females in each group (i.e., 6 males and females each in the LD group; 5 males and 6 females in the N-LD group). All subjects were native standard English speakers and demonstrated normal intelligence (IQ = 90 or above) based on their performance on the Slosson (1991) Intelligence Test–Revised. A *t* test revealed no significant differences between the subject groups on this measure of intelligence. Therefore, IQ was not used as a covariate in the data analysis procedures.

Subject selection criteria also included at least average language performance on several language measures. Language performance was evaluated on the basis of two measures of language comprehension and two measures of language production. Language comprehension was assessed using the Peabody Picture Vocabulary Test-Revised (PPVT; Dunn & Dunn, 1981), a test of single-word receptive vocabulary, and the Token Test-Part V (DeRenzi & Vignolo, 1962), a measure of sentence structure comprehension. Language production was assessed using the Vocabulary subtest of the Wechsler Adult Intelligence Scale (WAIS; Wechsler, 1955), a test of definitions, and an informal syntactic analysis of a spontaneous sample of conversational speech. The aim of the syntactic analysis was to ensure that all subjects had sufficient expressive structural language skills to generate a story. To be included as a subject, all participants were required to obtain scaled scores in the average or above range on the PPVT (i. e., scaled score = 85 or above), the WAIS Vocabulary subtest (i. e., scaled score = 7 or above), the Token Test (scaled score = 495 or above), and demonstrate intact expressive syntactic skills.

In addition, based on a questionnaire administered to each candidate, all subjects had unremarkable histories of primary sensory, physical, or emotional impairments.

A final subject selection criterion was educational background. All subjects had to have earned a minimum of a high school diploma (or equivalent) and a maximum of a baccalaureate degree. The occupations of the subjects varied a great deal and included homemaker, computer software company owner, salesperson, computer programmer, store manager, and secretary.

LD Subjects. The adults with learning disabilities were recruited from educational and social programs in the Washington, DC metropolitan area. It was recognized that a clear-cut diagnosis of LD would be difficult to ascertain or confirm in adults within the age range of interest in this study. As a result, potential subjects were required to meet at least one of two criteria: (a) had received a diagnosis of LD at some time during their school years, based on a significant discrepancy between IQ and achievement; and/or (b) had received special educational services during their school years.

N-LD Subjects. The N-LD subjects were recruited from PTAs of area public schools. These subjects had no history of language and learning problems, and had not received special education services during their school years. About one half of these adults completed post-high school education or skill training programs.

Procedure

All subjects were tested in one session in a quiet area of their homes. The subjects participated in two experimental story production tasks: story production to a picture and spontaneous story production. Following a prepared script, the examiner first introduced the story-to-picture task, and asked the subject to make up an original fictional story about a stimulus picture. The picture that was used was a theme-based black-and-white drawing and depicted three characters in a seemingly precarious situation on a lighthouse. A theme-based picture was selected because it does not lend itself to a simple listing or description of events as would an event-based picture.

Based on past experience with picture-elicitation tasks, it became apparent that when a single picture is presented to a subject, the subject assumes shared knowledge of the picture between him or herself and the examiner, even if explicitly told otherwise. It was found that this assumption of shared knowledge affects the manner in which stories are constructed (Roth & Spekman, 1990). To avoid this situation, a procedure was designed in which an easel was placed on the table in front of the subject. The easel was positioned to face the subject and was clearly out of the visual field of the examiner. The examiner placed three sealed envelopes on the table, each containing the "lighthouse" picture. The subject was told there were different pictures in each envelope and that the content of each particular envelope was unknown to the examiner. The subject was then instructed to select one envelope, remove the picture, and place it on the easel so that the examiner could not see the picture.

The second task involved spontaneous story production. Each subject was asked to make up a fictional story of his or her own. The order of task presentation was selected based on pilot data obtained from a small sample of adults. The adults in that sample (both LD and N-LD) were extremely reticent to participate in the story production tasks when the spontaneous story task was given first. They seemed more relaxed and were much more responsive when the session began with the picture task.

No time limit was imposed on either task. A predetermined set of prompts were used when a subject told a story that did not contain a resolution. A maximum of two prompts were given to each subject. The first prompt was a reminder to the subject that the story had to be "a complete story." If the subject still did not expand the tale to include a resolution, the second and final prompt was presented: "Could you tell me a little bit more about what happened?". All stories were audiotape recorded and later transcribed verbatim. If any doubt existed as to the inclusion of a story resolution, the prompt procedures were initiated. The head investigator subsequently listened to the tape and made the final decision regarding the end point of the story in question.

Interrater reliability checks were completed for each of the following procedures: (a) transcription, (b) proposition segmentation, (c) story grammar category assignment, (d) episode segmentation, (e) complete/incomplete episode identification, and (f) interepisode relation assignment. For each of these areas, one third of the stories told by the LD and N-LD subjects was reviewed by an independent observer who was trained in the specific procedures. An agreement was defined as an instance of congruence between raters prior to discussion. Percentage agreements were calculated separately for the LD and N-LD groups. This process yielded at least an 85% level of interrater agreement in each of the six reliability areas, with a range between 85% and 93%.

Following transcription, each story was segmented into propositions using Fillmore's (1968) definition. Each segmented story was then subjected to a story grammar analysis using Roth and Spekman's (1986) modified version of Stein and Glenn's (1979) story schema. Each proposition was coded into one of the seven story categories: (a) setting: information regarding character description and story context; (b) initiating event: occurrence that influences a character to act; (c) the character's response to these occurrences; (d) the plan made by the character to achieve the goal; (e) the overt attempt of the character to attain the goal; (f) the direct consequence of the overt actions; and (g) the character's reaction to the outcome.

In addition to the analysis of propositions in a story, each story was examined at the level of the episode. An episode is composed of propositions and is considered to be the basic building block of a story (Roth & Spekman, 1986). More specifically, an episode is a sequence of events that may include any or all of the seven categories occurring in the order just presented. Each story was divided into episodes and each episode was further classified as complete or incomplete. An episode was considered complete if it contained (a) a purpose in the form of either an initiating event or response; (b) an overt goal-directed behavior in the form of an attempt; and (c) a direct consequence indicating success or failure at attaining the goal (Stein & Glenn, 1979). Instances in which an attempt implied a consequence or resolution (e. g., "The man killed the bear") were also considered complete, despite the absence of an explicit direct consequence. An episode was considered incomplete when one or more of the essential components was not present.

The structure of episodes also was examined. This involved coding the types of story category information that were included in each episode.

A further area of interest was the manner in which successive episodes were connected to each other. To complete this analysis, the four kinds of interepisode relations identified by Stein and Glenn (1979) were used. A THEN relation was coded when the events in two episodes occurred successively in time but were not causally related. A CAUSE relation was coded when there was an explicitly stated causal relationship between the events in two succeeding episodes. An AND relation was coded when the events in two episodes occurred simultaneously. Finally, an EMBEDDED relation was coded when the events in an episode began after a previous episode was begun and terminated either before or at the same time as the previous episode.

Finally, the presence of story markers was recorded. This category included both beginning markers (i. e., *Once upon a time* or some variant) and ending markers (i. e., *The end* or some variant).

RESULTS

The results were examined from several different perspectives including story length, story category usage, episode integrity and structure, interepisode relations, and story markers and prompts. These areas were selected, in part, because they have been shown to be problematic for children and adolescents with learning disabilities. The data were analyzed using 2 (Group) × 2 (Task) analyses of variance with unequal *N*s. Vast differences in the length of stories produced by the subjects mandated the use of proportional data. Arcsine transformations were applied to the raw proportional data to achieve homogeneity of error variance (Kirk, 1968), yielding a homogeneous data set. The .05 level of significance was selected a priori as the error rate for each hypothesis. Post hoc analyses were conducted using the Neuman Keuls test. Several significant findings emerged from the data analysis procedures.

Length

Length of both stories and episodes was examined. Story length was defined as (a) the total number of propositions within a story, and (b) the mean number of episodes in a story. Episode length was operationalized as the total number of propositions contained in each episode. The findings showed that the stories told by the LD contained fewer propositions per story than those produced by the N-LD counterparts [$F(3, 44) = 4.68$, $p = .04$]. The average length of the LD stories was nearly 50 propositions ($SD = 34.2$) in comparison to almost 80 ($SD = 58.3$) for the average N-LD story. The number of propositions in a story also was related to task. For both groups, stories produced during the spontaneous story task were significantly longer than those generated on the picture task [$F(3, 44) = 4.28$, $p = .05$]. With respect to the number of episodes within stories, the results revealed no significant differences between the stories told by the LD and N-LD adults. On the average, stories contained between 5 and 6 episodes. A significant main effect for group was found, however, for episode length. The LD subjects produced episodes that contained substantially fewer propositions than the N-LD group [$F(3, 34) = 5.08$, $p = .03$]. Mean episode length was nearly 10 propositions ($SD = 3.1$) for the LD adults and almost 14 ($SD = 5.7$) for the N-LD subjects. Thus, these results indicate that both the stories and the episodes within stories generated by the LD subjects were shorter than those produced by their N-LD peers, but that both groups included an equivalent number of episodes in their stories.

Story Category Usage

In an effort to examine overall story content, a set of analyses was conducted to compare the proportional use of the seven different story categories (i. e., setting statements, initiating events, responses, plans, attempts, direct consequences, reactions; see Table 8.1). This analysis revealed that at least one third of the information in the stories told by both groups was setting information. Moreover, both subject groups spent minimal time setting up the conflict in stories (approximately 10%), describing the motivation of the protagonist (10%), or specifying the internal plans made to reach the goal (4%–7%). Substantially more time was spent describing the actual actions taken by the protagonist (22%–24%) and somewhat more time was spent indicating the ultimate resolution or

TABLE 8.1
Group Means and Standard Deviations of the Proportional Use of Story Category Types

	Group			
	LD		*N-LD*	
Category Type	*M*	*(SD)*	*M*	*(SD)*
Setting	34	(18)	33	(15)
Initiating event	10	(8)	11	(7)
Response	9	(8)	11	(9)
Plan	4	(6)	7	(9)
Attempt	22	(13)	24	(14)
Direct consequence[a]	15	(10)	9	(7)
Reaction	6	(5)	6	(6)

[a]Significant group difference at .05 level

consequence of the actions (approximately 12%). The only significant difference in proportional story category usage was direct consequences. The LD subjects produced proportionately more propositions containing direct consequence information than the N-LD counterparts [$F(3, 43) = 5.79$, $p = .02$].

Episode Integrity and Structure

Another focus of interest in this study was the episode. Although the mean number of episodes per story did not differentiate the subject groups, significant differences were found for episode integrity. *Episode integrity* was defined as the proportion of total episodes that were complete. As a group, the LD subjects produced a significantly lower proportion ($M = 22\%$, $SD = 22\%$) of complete episodes than the N-LD group [$M = 50\%$, $SD = 18\%$; $F(3, 44) = 20.0$, $p = .00$].

A complete episode was defined as containing an initiating event or response, an attempt, and a direct consequence. An episode was considered incomplete if it omitted one or more of the three key components. Analyses were conducted on the incomplete episodes to identify the kinds of information that were included and excluded from the stories (Table 8.2). For both groups, slightly more than half of the incomplete episodes contained initiating event information. Approximately half of the incomplete episodes of the LD adults and 80% of the N-LD subjects contained attempt information. Finally, direct consequence information was excluded from 60% of the incomplete episodes produced by the LD group and 84% of the N-LD group. Two of the three group comparisons were significant. First, a higher proportion of the incomplete episodes constructed by the LD subjects contained direct consequence statements than those generated by the N-LD group [$F(3, 44) = 6.59$, $p = .01$]. Second, the LD group produced a lower proportion of incomplete episodes that included at least one attempt statement

TABLE 8.2
Group Means and Standard Deviations for Proportion of Incomplete Episodes With Essential Story Category Information

	Group			
	LD		*N-LD*	
Story Category	*M*	*(SD)*	*M*	*(SD)*
Initiating event	53	(32)	55	(38)
Attempt	53	(36)	80	(29)
Direct consequence	40	(31)	17	(29)

than the N-LD counterparts. This was true only on the picture story task [$F(3, 44) = 4.71$, $p = .04$].

Episode structure was measured by calculating the proportion of episodes (complete and incomplete combined) that contained one or more proposition in each story grammar category. The results revealed no significant group or task differences and no interaction effects for any of the story categories.

Interepisode Relations

Another aspect of story production explored in this study was the manner in which episodes were connected to one another. This information was obtained by calculating the proportion of total interepisode relations that were of each of the four different types. The ANOVA results showed significant group differences for CAUSE relations and THEN relations. The LD subjects used proportionately fewer [$M = 1\%$, $SD = .03\%$; $F(3, 43) = 12.669$; $p = .001$] causal linkages than the N-LD group [$M = 15\%$, $SD = 18\%$; $F(3, 43) = 9.583$, $p = .003$]. In contrast, THEN relations were used proportionately more frequently by the LD subjects to connect their episodes than by the N-LD group ($M = 95\%$, $SD = 18\%$ for LD; $M = 71\%$, $SD = 28\%$ for N-LD). No significant group or task differences and no interactions were found for AND and EMBEDDED relations.

Story Markers and Prompts

The final aspects of the analysis procedures involved the adults' use of story markers and the tester's need to use prompts to elicit complete stories from the adult subjects. The story marker analysis revealed no significant main effects or interaction effects. The analysis of prompts yielded significant main effects for group and task and a significant interaction effect [$F(3, 44) = 5.42$, $p = .03$]. Examination of these findings indicates that a higher mean number of prompts were given to the LD subjects in the story to picture task than to the N-LD group ($M = .50$, $SD = .66$ for LD; $M = .10$, $SD = .30$ for N-LD).

DISCUSSION

The results of the present study provide preliminary outcome information regarding a specific area of narrative discourse development in adults with learning disabilities. The oral story production performance of the learning disabled adults studied here suggests three things: (a) LD adults possess knowledge of basic story structure and can apply that knowledge in the production of oral stories; (b) there seems to be growth in certain aspects of story production with increased age; and, (c) some differences in oral narration abilities may persist into adulthood in this population.

First, the stories produced by the adults with learning disabilities conformed to the basic rules of story grammar. They constructed stories that contained orderly event sequences, evidenced use of all seven types of story category information, and generated at least some episodes that were structurally complete. This fundamental knowledge of story structure (i. e., narrative schema) also was demonstrated by the young adolescents studied by Roth and Spekman (1986). Thus, it appears that once acquired, narrative schema continues to be used as a framework for organizing and presenting story information.

Second, the story production performance of the adults in this study indicates that narrative discourse skills may undergo improvement between early adolescence and adulthood. A comparison of our sample of LD adolescents (Roth & Spekman, 1986) and the adults studied here shows growth in two facets of story production: the structure of episodes and task effects on story production performance. Although the adult and adolescent subjects were not matched samples, they had similar backgrounds and characteristics with respect to IQ levels, socioeconomic status, native and primary language, and lack of comorbid conditions.

With respect to episode structure, recall that the young adolescents with learning disabilities were found to omit the entire middle sections of an episode. Proportionately fewer of their episodes contained response, attempt, and plan statements than their normally achieving (NA) counterparts. This pattern of episode structure was not displayed by the adult LD sample. In fact, there were no significant differences between the LD and N-LD groups in the proportional use of any of the story grammar categories within an episode.

This finding indicates that some difficulties with episode structure may diminish over time and become resolved in the adult years. By adulthood, then, individuals with a history of learning disabilities may become more aware of and more able to include information regarding attitudes and motivations of the main character, as well as cognitive planning and overt actions of the protagonist to obtain the desired end. The inclusion of these kinds of essential story information may reflect growth in role-taking skills, that is, an improved ability of the adult speaker to take the perspective of the listener in determining shared knowledge and listener needs. Roth and Spekman hypothesized that their adolescent LD subjects were aware of the importance of key story information (because their stories contained instances of all of the different types of story information), but did not convey this information linguistically on a consistent basis. The authors concluded that the stories of the LD adolescents resembled those of developmentally younger children. The behavior of the adult sample may reflect the completion of a developmental process. The apparent improvement seen in the episode structure of the adult LD subjects may also, in part, simply reflect their greater life experience with feelings, setting goals, making plans, and the like.

The other area of narrative improvement found in this study involved the effects of different elicitation tasks on story production performance. When Roth and Spekman (1989a) compared the storytelling performance of their LD adolescents on a spontaneous versus story-to-picture task, they found that the LD students derived benefit from the structure provided by the picture stimulus. The stories they produced in response to the picture were more complete and better organized than their spontaneously generated narratives. In contrast, the performance of the NA group was not affected by the picture, and remained consistent across elicitation conditions.

The results of the present study show that the adults with learning disabilities behaved similarly to the nondisabled adults in that they performed equally well on both tasks. Like the nondisabled adults, the elicitation task had very little effect on the structure of their stories. Both groups produced longer stories in the spontaneous production task. The only measurable LD–N-LD group differentiator was that the LD adults were given more prompts during the picture task. The consistency of performance across tasks may reflect a more firmly developed sense of story, a greater degree of confidence or experience with the narrative form or a combination of these and other factors.

Despite the positive changes in story production found in this study, the findings also indicate that oral narration is an aspect of language that continues to pose problems for individuals with learning disabilities. The results show some continued significant differences between the oral story production abilities of adults with and without learning disabilities. The main areas of the persistent difference involved length, episode integrity, and interepisode relations. The stories and the episodes produced by the LD adults were significantly shorter and contained fewer units of meaning than those generated by the N-LD group. Although length was a significant group differentiator, it is important to recognize that length itself is not a sensitive indicator of overall story quality. For example, one LD subject's spontaneous story was quite short (containing only 20 propositions), yet, charmingly recounted the antics of a magical cat named Fritz who had the power to turn himself into any object or person that suited his fancy. In contrast, a much longer spontaneous story produced by another LD subject (consisting of 94 propositions) involved a laborious and repetitive portrayal of the childhood activities of a fictional girl named Stephanie. These examples clearly show that overall story length is a variable that cannot be viewed in isolation, but one that must be considered in relation to other aspects of story structure. With this in mind, it is notable that there may be a developmental increase in story length as a function of increased age. The stories produced by Roth and Spekman's LD and NA adolescent subjects averaged 37 and 54 propositions, respectively, in comparison to 50 and 80 propositions for the respective groups of LD and N–LD adults.

More significant than story length may be the length of episodes within stories. Recall that the findings showed that episode integrity differentiated the groups. Similar to the young adolescents, the stories told by the LD adults contained a significantly lower proportion of complete episodes than those produced by the nondisabled group. To be considered complete, an episode must contain certain information that is most usually expressed in at least three propositions. Complete episodes typically must contain a minimum of three propositions. For this reason, the length of an episode may be related to its completeness or integrity.

Episode integrity has been shown to be a meaningful basis for the comparison of story structure. Story structure analysis at the level of the episode was first pursued by Roth and Spekman (1986). At that time, the authors speculated that the episode represents a higher hierarchical unit of story structure than does the individual proposition, and therefore can be considered the basic building block of stories. In the present study, only 20% of the episodes constructed by the LD adults were complete in comparison to 50% for the N-LD group. Clearly, the presence of some incomplete episodes in a story would not necessarily interrupt the flow of the story. But, when many of the episodes are incomplete, plot lines are left unresolved and may result in a great deal of listener confusion.

The precise reason for the diminished use of complete episodes by the LD subjects is not clear. It may reflect one aspect of the cyclical nature of learning disabilities as a life-long condition. We know that reading is an activity that continues to be difficult for adults with learning disabilities. Studies have repeatedly documented severe and chronic reading deficits on standardized tests of academic achievement (e.g., Spekman et al., 1992). This persistent struggle with reading is highlighted by the results of a survey conducted by Fafard and Haubrich (1981), in which reading was one of four areas identified as "most difficult" by a sample of LD adults. One impact of their reading problems may be that they do not enjoy the reading process and do not routinely engage in reading as a source of pleasure or entertainment. Or it may be that they read, but their preferred reading materials do not consist of novels or other storylike material. Over time, their exposure to literature may be quite restricted, and consequently, their knowledge or awareness of story structure is not activated or reinforced on an ongoing basis.

Interestingly, the stories told by the adolescent group contained higher proportions of complete episodes than those generated by the adults. This was true for both ability groups. Sixty percent of the episodes produced by the LD adolescents were complete, as were almost 80% of those generated by the NA peers, in contrast to the 20% and 50%, respectively, for the adult subjects. One explanation for this seemingly surprising outcome is that narratives are a primary focus in current educational curricula. As such, students in the primary and secondary grades receive repeated and explicit instruction on narrative construction in both oral and written language domains. Such instruction includes structured assignments, teacher-monitored editing, and verbal feedback. This emphasis may result in a higher level of awareness of and adherence to the components of a complete story than the adult who does not have this kind of didactic formal exposure to narrative structure. The adults may have not lost the ability, per se, but it may not be at a level of conscious awareness.

The final aspect of oral narration in which significant group differences were found involved interepisode relations. The adults with learning disabilities relied more heavily on THEN relations to connect episodes within their stories than the adults without learning disabilities. Although the THEN relation was used most frequently by both subject groups, the LD adults utilized this relation type almost exclusively (i.e., 95%). The nondisabled adults employed the THEN relation far less frequently (i.e., 71%) to join episodes. The THEN relation is considered the most basic kind of episode connector because it simply links event sequences that occur successively in time. It is roughly equivalent to the conjunction "and then."

The CAUSE relation was used proportionately more often by the N-LD adults than by the LD group, whose total use of this relation approximated 1%. CAUSE relations connect episodes in which there is a direct cause–effect relationship between two plot sequences, and are therefore viewed as more sophisticated episode connectors than THEN relations. Causality represents a complex cognitive construct. Specification of causality between episodes requires a greater degree of planning and cognitive maturity on the part of the narrator than does the simple linear sequencing of events.

The EMBEDDED relation is the most complex interepisode linkage. Like CAUSE relations, embedded episodes also require a significant amount of planning on the part of the narrator. However, they further necessitate the ability to organize at least two plot sequences simultaneously and coordinate them into a cohesive story unit. Although EMBEDDED relations did not reach statistical significance in this study, two points are worthy of note. First, embedded episodes occurred only in the story-to-picture task; there were no instances of this relation type in spontaneous stories. Second, EMBEDDED relations constituted only 1% of the interepisode linkages used by the LD adults, whereas the N-LD adults utilized the EMBEDDED linkage much more frequently (11%).

The pattern of interepisode relation usage exhibited by the LD adults in this study is strikingly similar to that previously displayed by the adolescent LD group. Thus, it appears that differences persist between LD and N-LD groups in the linguistic strategies that are used to connect episodes within stories. LD adults may continue to rely more predominantly on linkage devices that place fewer demands on the cognitive system and that are linguistically less sophisticated.

CONCLUSIONS AND DIRECTIONS FOR FUTURE RESEARCH

The structure of the stories told by the LD adults indicate that they had more difficulty with oral narration than the N-LD adults. The specific kinds of narrative behaviors that differentiated the LD and N-LD adults involved reduced story and episode length, the completeness of episodes in stories, and the use of less sophisticated linguistic markers for connecting episodes to one another.

Our findings also suggest that certain differences with narrative discourse may persist into adulthood, whereas others may change across the life span. A comparison of the present findings with those reported previously (Roth & Spekman, 1986) on a sample of young adolescents with LD indicate that improvement may occur in the overall structure of episodes and in the consistency of oral story production performance across different tasks.

This study represents a first attempt to gather outcome information regarding the narrative discourse skills of adults with and without a history of learning disabilities. It focused on one narrative discourse process: oral story production. Moreover, the analysis procedures used involved a story grammar approach. Although a story grammar analysis provides important information regarding the structural organization of stories, it should not be viewed as the sole measure of story intactness and structure. There are aspects of stories that are not revealed using a story structure approach, but that may affect overall story quality. These include functional aspects such as character development and the use of more intricate plot sequences, as well as structural aspects such as the syntactic integrity of stories and the adequate use of linguistic cohesion to tie sentences together in stories to form a textual whole.

Factors such as these warrant further attention, not only because they contribute to story construction, but also because children and young adolescents with LD have been shown to demonstrate difficulties in these areas of language. For example, Roth, Spekman, and Fye (in press) were interested in the reference cohesion patterns in stories told by young LD adolescents, because a key aspect of successful narration involves the ability to make clear reference to characters, places, and things in stories. The results showed that the LD group had problems using reference cohesion as a linguistic tool for organizing and unifying their stories. They exhibited problems with the correct use of cohesive markers and demonstrated ambiguous reference usage. This pattern of use created discontinuity in their stories and decreased the internal coherence of their narratives. There is some evidence that LD adults also have problems with linguistic cohesion in the written language domain. Hoy and Gregg (1992) reported that their group of LD adults displayed a vague and ambiguous use of cohesive devices in written language samples.

Given these findings, it appears that narrative processing is a fertile and promising area of inquiry in the adult LD population. Because story narration is not a unitary construct, future research should focus on a variety of different processing modalities, including memory and comprehension, and in both the oral and written language domains. This kind of comprehensive approach will result in a clearer understanding of the narrative discourse systems of adults with learning disabilities.

REFERENCES

Blalock, J. (1982). Persistent auditory language deficits in adults with learning disabilities. *Journal of Learning Disabilities, 15*, 604–609.

Blalock, J. W. (1987). Problems in mathematics. In D. J. Johnson & J. W. Blalock (Eds.), *Adults with learning disabilities: Clinical studies* (pp. 205–217). New York: Grune & Stratton.

Buchanan, M., & Wolf, S. (1986). A comprehensive study of learning disabled adults. *Journal of Learning Disabilities, 19*, 34–38.

Chesler, B. (1982). ACLD vocational committee survey on LD adults. *ACLD Newsbrief*, No. 145.

Crais, E. R., & Chapman, R. S. (1987). Story recall and inferencing in language/learning-disabled children and non-disabled children. *Journal of Speech and Hearing Disorders, 52*, 50–55.

Cronin, M. E., & Patton, J. R. (in press). *Life skills for students with special needs: A guide for developing real life programs.* Austin, TX: PRO-ED.

DeRenzi, E., Vignolo, L. A. (1962). The DeRenzi Token Test: A sensitive test to detect receptive disturbances in aphasics. *Brain, 85*, 556–578.

Dunn, L. M., & Dunn, L. M. (1981). *Peabody Picture Vocabulary Test–Revised.* Circle Pines, MN:American Guidance Service.

Fafard, M., & Haubrich, P. A. (1981). Vocational and social adjustment of learning disabled young adults: A followup study. *Learning Disability Quarterly, 4*, 122–130.

Fillmore, C. (1968). The case for case. In F. Bach & R. Harms (Eds.), *Universals in linguistic theory* (pp. 1–90). New York: Holt, Rinehart & Winston.

Graybeal, C. (1981). Memory for stories in language impaired children. *Applied Psycholinguistics, 2*, 269–283.

Gregg, N., & Hoy, C. (1990). Referencing: The cohesive use of pronouns in the written narratives of college underprepared writers, nondisabled writers, and writers with learning disabilities. *Journal of Learning Disabilities, 9*, 557–563.

Hansen, C. L. (1978). Story retelling used with average and learning disabled readers as a measure of reading comprehension. *Learning Disability Quarterly, 1*, 62–69.

Haring, K. A., Lovett, D. L., & Smith, D. D. (1990). A follow-up study of recent special education graduates of learning disabilities programs. *Journal of Learning Disabilities, 23*, 108–113.

Hoffmann, F. J., Sheldon, K. L., Minskoff, E. H., Sautter, S. W., Stiedle, E. F., Baker, D. P., & Bailey, M. B. (1987). Needs of learning disabled adults. *Journal of Learning Disabilities, 20*, 43–52.

Johnson, D. J. (1987a). Reading disabilities. In D. J. Johnson & J. W. Blalock (Eds.), *Adults with learning disabilities: Clinical studies* (pp. 145–171). New York: Grune & Stratton.

Johnson, D. J. (1987b). Disorders of written language. In D. J. Johnson & J. W. Blalock (Eds.), *Adults with learning disabilities: Clinical studies* (pp. 173–203). New York: Grune & Stratton.

Kirk, R. E. (1968). *Experimental design: Procedures for the behavioral sciences.* Belmont, CA: Brooks/Cole.

La Greca, A. M. (1987). Children with learning disabilities: Interpersonal skills and social competence. *Journal of Reading, Writing, and Learning Disabilities International, 3*, 167–185.

Merritt, D. D., & Liles, B. Z. (1987). Story grammar ability in children with and without language disorder: Story generation, story retelling, and story comprehension. *Journal of Speech and Hearing Research, 20*, 529–542.

Oakhill, J. (1984). Inferential and memory skills in children's comprehension of stories. *Journal of Educational Psychology, 54*, 31–39.

Patton, J. R., & Palloway, E. A. (1992). Learning disabilities: The challenges of adulthood. *Journal of Learning Disabilities, 25*, 410–415.

Rogan, L. L., & Hartman, L. D. (1990). Adult outcome of learning disabled students ten years after initial follow-up. *Learning Disabilities Focus, 5*, 91–102.

Roth, F. P., & Spekman, N. J. (1986). Narrative discourse: Spontaneously-generated stories of learning-disabled and normally achieving students. *Journal of Speech and Hearing Disorders, 51*, 8–23.

Roth, F. P., & Spekman, N. J. (1989a). *Narrative discourse proficiency of learning disabled students: Differences in elicitation procedures.* Symposium for Research in Child Language Disorders, Madison, WI.

Roth, F. P., & Spekman, N. J. (1989b). Oral syntactic proficiency of learning disabled students: A spontaneous speech sampling analysis. *Journal of Speech and Hearing Research, 32*, 67–77.

Roth, F. P., & Spekman, N. J.(1990). *Reference cohesion in written stories of learning disabled students.* Paper presented at the American Speech-Language-Hearing Association, Seattle, WA.

Roth, F. P., Spekman, N. J., & Fye, E. C. (in press). Reference cohesion in the oral narratives of learning disabled and normally achieving students. *Learning Disabilities Quarterly.*

Silver, L. (1984). *The joy of learning should not be a nightmare: The emotional problems faced by individuals with learning disabilities.* Paper presented at the Dian Ridenour Memorial Lecture Series, Evanston, IL.

Slosson, R. L. (1991). *Slosson Intelligence Test-Revised.* Los Angeles, CA: Western Psychological Services.

Spekman, N. J., Goldberg, R. J., & Herman, K. L. (1992). Learning disabled children grow up: A search for factors related to success in the young adult years. *Learning Disabilities: Research and Practice, 7*, 161–170.

Stein, N., & Glenn, C. (1979). An analysis of story comprehension in elementary school children. In R. O. Freedle (Ed.), *New directions in discourse processing* (pp. 53–120). Norwood, NJ: Ablex.

Vaughn, S. R., & La Greca, A. M. (1988). Social interventions for learning disabilities. In K. A. Kavale (Ed.), *Learning disabilities: State of the art in practice* (pp. 123–140), Austin, TX: PRO-ED.

Wechsler, D. (1955). *Wechsler Adult Intelligence Scale.* San Antonio, TX: Psychological Corporation.

Westby, C. E. (1982). Cognitive and linguistic aspects of children's narrative development. *Communication Disorders, 7*, 1–16.

Worden, P., Malmgren, L., & Gabourie, P. (1982). Memory for stories in learning disabled adults. *Journal of Learning Disabilities, 15*, 145–151.

Worden, P., & Nakamura, G. (1982). Story comprehension and recall in learning disabled versus normal college students. *Journal of Educational Psychology, 74*, 633–641.

Zigmond, N., & Thornton, H. (1985). Follow-up of post-secondary age learning disabled graduates and drop-outs. *Learning Disabilities Research, 1*, 50–55.

Chapter 9

Studies of Discourse Production in Adults With Alzheimer's Disease

Jonathan S. Ehrlich
Pro-Speech, Somerset, NJ

The language abilities of adults with dementia of Alzheimer's type (DAT) have come under increasing scrutiny in the cognitive neurosciences. The bulk of research to date suggests that language skills deteriorate in DAT over time in a characteristic manner with semantic and some pragmatic aspects of language far more vulnerable to impairment than syntax and phonology. Most studies have addressed issues of semantic–lexical processing, and have not focused on discourse, or language that extends beyond the sentence level.

This chapter discusses recent research on the discourse production of DAT adults and focuses on narrative discourse. The rationale for examining discourse of DAT adults is considered in light of a review of specific studies of their discourse performance. Some of the methodological problems associated with this area of investigation are highlighted. Specific questions are raised about the influence of the type of task and the number of variables being examined in experimental studies. Finally, suggestions for future studies of discourse examination of DAT adults are explored.

DISCOURSE DEFICITS IN DAT

The language production deficits in DAT adults show several consistent features and patterns. This clinical picture includes semantic paraphasias (Bayles, 1982), a reduced vocabulary (Hier, Hagenlocker, & Shindler, 1985), a marked deficit on confrontation naming (Martin & Fedio, 1983), and repetitiveness, tangentiality, and the use of indefinite terms in discourse (Horner, Heyman, Kanter, Royall, & Aker, 1983; Obler, 1983). There is also evidence that syntax and phonology are relatively more preserved than semantic and lexical components of language (Bayles & Boone, 1982; Irigaray, 1973; Kempler, Curtiss, & Jackson, 1987; Obler, 1983; Schwartz, Marin, & Saffran, 1979; Whitaker, 1976).

The study of the language functions of DAT adults has been fueled in part by the knowledge that the behavioral pathology associated with cerebral dysfunction can reveal the workings of the normal state. Thus, the language deficits of DAT can be viewed as a source of evidence about the relationship between nonlinguistic cognitive abilities (e.g., attention, memory) and language processing (Obler, 1981, 1983). Obler (1983), for one, claimed that a semantic deficit underlies the language pathology of DAT adults. For example, the lack of specificity in lexical selection and the misuse of syntactic items that carry more semantic burden (e.g., "before," "because") is attributed to an impairment of semantic processing.

Bayles and Kaszniak (1987), in contrast, interpreted the language data of DAT adults within a framework of information processing and memory, and suggest that decreased ideation is at the heart of dementia. Semantic memory, which forms part of the "central" or nonmodular system, consists of "knowledge of the world abstractly coded" and inferential processes. Semantic memory has a characteristic breakdown in dementia according to this interpretation. Bayles and Kaszniak claimed that a progressive impairment to the contents and processes of semantic memory accounts for the communication impairment in DAT. *Semantic memory*, as used by Bayles and Kaszniak here, should be distinguished from the more narrow sense of *semantic processing* cited by Obler (1983). Semantic memory incorporates language and nonlanguage knowledge, whereas semantic processing relates to linguistic knowledge of meaning and reference. This distinction implies different sources for the language errors of DAT adults.

The neuropathology in DAT, relative to a focal lesion, is diffuse and includes neurofibrillary tangles, neuritic plaques, granulovacuolar degeneration, and brain atrophy; this pathology often involves the temporal lobes including hippocampal structures (Bayles & Kaszniak, 1987). The study of the language deterioration of DAT adults may eventually provide support for different neural models of language organization in the brain.

Discourse abilities of adults with acquired cerebral pathology have come under closer examination in the last decade. *Discourse* is defined here as naturally occurring language that extends beyond the sentence level or across sentences. This review broadly considers the discourse of DAT adults and then focuses on narrative discourse, which is one genre of discourse. *Narrative*, for the purposes of this chapter, is a unit of language consisting of several propositions that collectively represent several events, as in a story. This form of discourse is distinguished from conversational discourse or dialogue.

The application of discourse study to adult neurogenic communication disorders properly begins with aphasia. Studies of the comprehension and production of discourse in aphasia, which are reviewed elsewhere in this volume, support the claim that the global features of discourse organization are relatively more preserved in aphasia than the linguistic components such as lexical and syntactic processing (Ulatowska, Freedman-Stern, Weiss-Doyel, Macaluso-Haynes, & North, 1983; Ulatowska, North, & Macaluso-Haynes, 1981).

In recent years, researchers and clinicians have recognized the important role that pragmatic or extralinguistic contextual variables play in normal and pathological communication behavior. The analysis of discourse production, which as a task is close to naturalistic communication, is thus gaining support as clinically relevant for brain-damaged adults. For example, Davis and Wilcox (1985) offered an interactive model of aphasia rehabilitation based on a pragmatic orientation in which conversational abilities are fostered.

The discourse abilities in DAT adults deteriorate in a characteristic way (Bayles, 1986; Hier et al., 1985; Horner et al., 1983; Irigaray, 1973; Nicholas, Obler, Albert, & Helm-Estabrooks, 1985; Obler, 1981) and may be marked by fewer substantives, more circumlocutions and digressions from the topic. This profile of "empty" speech in discourse, is also characteristically egocentric and concrete with ideational perseverations, and either excessive speech or little or no speech in the late stages.

A key contribution to our understanding of DAT and language behavior is the identification of several stages of discourse changes (Horner et al., 1983; Obler, 1983). In early stages of DAT, a mild discourse deficit occurs with elaborate speech and occasional repetition of ideas although discourse generally remains on topic; there is also a mild word-finding difficulty and responses to questions are not precise. In the middle stages of the disease, a moderate deficit in discourse evolves into more frequent repetition and revision of ideas, paragrammatisms, a decrease in the amount of information relative to the amount of talk, and more self-referential comments. At the late stages of DAT, more severe deficits in discourse emerge. The connected language of DAT adults becomes increasingly cluttered with repetitions, revisions, and intrusions. There is further reduction in the number of ideas expressed as well as increased difficulty maintaining a stream of thought. A decreased mean length of utterance (MLU) and excessive speech or failure to initiate talk are also characteristic of the later stages of DAT. Finally, there is also violation of turn-taking rules in conversation.

Several recent studies that focus on narrative discourse abilities in DAT adults are examined in more detail. Shekim and LaPointe (1984) attempted to "quantitatively describe aspects of discourse" of 9 DAT and 9 normal adults through several elicited narrative discourses: picture story description, telling a memorable story, expository or subject-oriented discourse, and procedural discourse or telling how something is done. They looked at cohesion, based on Halliday and Hasan's (1976) system, performance deviations (e.g., incomplete utterances), length of communication unit (CU), which is identical to Loban's (1976) T-unit, rate of speech, and percentage of maze words. A *maze* was defined as a series of words (or initial parts of words) or unattached fragments that do not constitute a communication unit. The DAT adults were found to have fewer cohesive ties per CU, more exophora or references to information outside of the text, more performance deviations, slower speech rate, and more maze words. The length of CU when mazes were removed was not significantly different for groups. Speech rate correlated negatively with the severity of dementia and the percentage of maze words correlated positively with the duration of dementia.

Santo Pietro and Berman (1984) examined the narrative discourse of a group of institutionalized elderly adults with and without senile dementia. Subjects were categorized on the basis of their performance on the Mental Status Questionnaire into severe, moderate, mild, or no impairment groups, which included a sample of 8 men and 64 women with a mean age of 82.8. The Cookie Theft picture description task from the Boston Diagnostic Aphasia Examination (Goodglass & Kaplan, 1983) was administered and Yorkston and Beukelman's (1980) content analysis procedure was used to quantify the amount and efficiency of information imparted. They reported significant differences in the number of content units only between the groups with severe and no impairment. Not surprisingly, high negative correlations were noted between the amount of content and efficiency measures and the severity of dementia. However, unlike the study of Shekim and La Pointe, syllables per minute or speech rate did not significantly differentiate among the groups. Overall, the more demented subjects conveyed less meaning than the unimpaired subjects. Santo Pietro and Berman (1984) also noted the presence of more egocentric references, fillers, and nonspecific words in the narratives of the demented subjects.

The Cookie Theft picture description task was also used by Hier et al. (1985), along with other language measures in their study comparing the language production abilities of adults with Alzheimer's disease, stroke-related dementia (SRD), and normal controls. Although subject selection was more careful in respect to etiology than in Santo Pietro and Berman (1984), the influence of age was not controlled. DAT adults were significantly older than the SRD subjects, and no exact age data were reported for the healthy controls except that they were older than 59. Hier and his colleagues measured a broad range of language variables from the elicited discourses that included number of words, number of unique words, MLU, percentage of prepositional phrases and subordinate clauses, empty words, palilalia, phrasal perseveration, information units drawn from the picture content, and sentence fragments. They found reductions in all language variables, although lexical deficits were more pronounced than syntactic ones. In the picture description task, all demented subjects used fewer total and unique words, fewer prepositional phrases and subordinate clauses, more sentence fragments, and fewer relevant observations of the narrative content than the controls. DAT subjects in the early stages were found to resemble Anomic aphasics, and in the more advanced stages, presented as Wernicke's and Transcortical sensory aphasics. Hier et al. related this later finding to a dissolution of the "mental lexicon." They also considered the decrease in relevant observations to reflect a general intellectual decline rather than a disorder specific to language. Similarly, they attributed aposiopesis (interruption of sentences in midsentence) to a nonlinguistic deficit in that "the dementia subject fails to perceive a necessity to complete utterances" (p. 128).

Beeson, Bayles, Tomoeda, and Slauson (1987) elicited picture description narratives from 15 mild DAT patients (3.7 on the Global Deterioration Scale—GDS), 20 moderate DAT patients (5.5 on the GDS), 15 fluent and nonfluent aphasics, and 26 normal elderly controls. Two Rockwell pictures ("Easter Morning" and "The Homecoming") served as the stimuli and response measures included the number of words, number of information units (new relevant pieces of information), and story content that was further scored for 12 observations concerning setting (character, time, or place), events (action or state), and gist (theme), with 6 of the 12 observations considered "inferential" by the researchers. Only the moderate DAT and nonfluent aphasic groups had significantly fewer words in their narratives than the mild DAT, fluent aphasic and normal control subjects; however, there were significantly fewer information units for the mild and moderate DAT and the nonfluent groups than for the control and the fluent aphasic groups. There were fewer event than setting observations for the disorder groups, and fewer gist and inferential observations for the mild DAT, nonfluent aphasic, and moderate DAT groups. Similar to the Shekim and La Pointe results, mental status correlated highly with the content measures that Beeson et al. claimed reflects "the cognitive demands of the narrative task" (p. 8). Beeson and her colleagues conclude that information units are sensitive measures to group differences.

Selected discourse features in the language production of six senile DAT and six normal elderly adults were also examined by Ripich and Terrell (1988). Samples of dialogic discourse were elicited through topic-directed interviews and analyzed for the number of words, amount of turn-taking, patterns of propositional forms (complete, incomplete, or nonpropositions), cohesion (appropriate and inappropriate), and the listener perceptions of the coherence or plausibility of the propositions. The DAT adults were found to use many more words and conversational turns than the elderly controls. The number of propositions (*proposition* was defined as an argument plus its relations) did not statistically differentiate between the DAT and normal adults, although the DAT adults had a higher percentage of incomplete propositions (e.g., "My husband he had a . . . we were there"). Similarly, inappropriate use of cohesion was higher in the DAT group, but not to a statistically significant degree. The omission of a referent as in the example just cited was a more common error for the DAT adults. Trained listeners judged the discourses of all subjects for incoherence or inappropriateness and found no such instances in the normal adults' discourses; 11 out of 1,733 propositions of the DAT adults were found to be incoherent. The authors do not cite any statistical differences between groups for this variable. However, they state that multiple influences may be involved in coherent discourse; they suggest that the speaker's ability to take the perspective of the listener as well as the listener's ability to predict the speaker's message are essential ingredients to discourse coherence. They speculate that "The missing elements in the speech of SDAT patients may reflect a breakdown in a process of discourse, namely the ability of the speaker to take the perspective of the listener" (p. 14).

Ulatowska et al. (1988) investigated the discourse performance of DAT adults across a range of tasks such as retelling a story, detailing a procedure, describing a pictured story, and providing a summary. The DAT subjects relative to the normal controls were more prone to include fewer target propositions in the picture story task and more irrelevant steps in the procedures; they also produced more incomplete sentences and showed an abundance of reference errors such as a higher proportion of pronouns to nouns and more demonstratives or deictic terms. However, there were no differences in the amount of language produced, which was described in terms of T-units, length of T-units and clauses. The DAT subjects also included the essential superstructural elements to the story tasks (e.g., setting, participants). Also, similar to the findings of Ripich and Terrell (1988), a group of listeners was not able to discriminate the DAT from normal subjects.

A picture story task was also used by Smith, Chenery, and Murdoch (1989) to examine a group of 18 DAT subjects in their semantic and syntactic abilities. These subjects, who had a mean age of 82.5 years, were considered to be in the moderate to moderate–severe stages of dementia. Subjects described the picture from the Western Aphasia Battery and a Yorkston and Beukelman (1980) analysis of narrative content was applied. The DAT subjects were found to use shorter phrases and required more time to impart the target information in the picture story; that is they were less efficient than the normal controls. However, there were no significant group differences for the number of content units or target substantives, syllables, and the syllables per minute index. According to the authors, this somewhat unexpected finding that the DAT subjects provided the same amount of information as the normal controls is related to the complexity of the picture stimulus. Smith et al. suggested that picture story tasks "that require a holistic integration of linguistic and nonlinguistic information at the conceptual or message level representation" (p. 539) would be more difficult for the DAT adults than picture stimuli that depict details and events that are not necessarily integrated. The more complex stimuli should result in reduced content for DAT adults. They also claimed that DAT adults are impaired in their ability to map "functional structure roles at an appropriately complex phrasal level" (p. 540).

Ulatowska and Bond (1990) examined the narrative performance of DAT subjects on a sequential picture task with four and seven picture stimuli; these stimuli contained one episode per panel. The DAT subjects had more narrative disruption in the seven picture condition. However, Ulatowska and Bond did not control for the amount of content between the two conditions. It is likely that the seven picture condition entailed more content and greater complexity than the single picture condition.

Taken together, these studies show several consistent features of narrative discourse deviations for DAT adults. Across a range of tasks such as describing a picture, telling how to do something, and talking about a topic, the DAT adults show limitations in the use of cohesion and expression of content. Their discourses contain more exophora, or references to information outside of the text, more mazes or sentence fragments, fewer unique words, and less syntactic complexity when compared with the discourse of the normal elderly. An increase in the number of words was reported only in the topic oriented discourses of DAT adults (Ripich & Terrell, 1988). The volume of discourse produced may be more a function of the type of task and less one of the disorder.

METHODOLOGICAL AND THEORETICAL IMPLICATIONS

It is instructive at this point to review some of the methodological problems regarding the study of the discourse of dementia. Many of the applied discourse studies discussed previously are descriptive and lack experimental control. For example, memory difficulty, one of the hallmarks of DAT, is not controlled for in Bayles (1982), in which a story-retelling task was used. Shekim and LaPointe (1984) also used several memory-laden tasks, such as telling a memorable story. The amount and complexity of information in the picture stimuli is also not well controlled. Although Beeson et al., (1987) came closest to specifying the amount of content in their narrative tasks, they did not directly manipulate this variable. Finally, there are often too many dependent variables reported, as in Shekim and LaPointe (1984), Hier et al. (1985), and Ripich and Terrell (1988) to allow valid inferences. Because multiple comparisons are made, the likelihood of finding differences due to chance is increased. Perhaps, the use of more stringent alpha levels or other corrective procedures would improve the accuracy of the statistics.

Another problem in discourse study is the low reliability engendered by using too few narrative tasks. Given the documented inter- and intrasubject variation in discourse production, the representativeness of the specific discourse behaviors might be questioned. That is, the discourse behaviors being measured should show some consistency.

There also may be some question about the accuracy of the diagnosis of DAT. The diagnostic criteria for probable Alzheimer's dementia as suggested by the NINCDS-ADRDA Work Group (McKhann et al., 1984) are not always explicitly followed. Consequently, subjects displaying more focal neurological deficits such as those found in multi-infarct dementia as well as other dementing conditions may cloud the picture of language deterioration in DAT.

Some basic methodological issues confronting the study of the discourse of dementia have been identified. This discussion now shifts to one of several theoretical issues relating to the disourse of dementia. Changes in discourse production such as digressions from the topic and ideational perseveration have long been considered by many researchers and clinicians to be reliable features in the communicative pathology of DAT adults.

The review presented here of recent research centering on the narrative discourse abilities of DAT adults reveals a reduced ability to convey meaning and make relevant observations; more nonspecific words and fewer unique words are produced in oral narrative tasks such as describing a picture. Although there is general agreement concerning the occurrence of these characteristics in DAT adults, an explanation of these narrative features in terms of the linguistic and cognitive deficits in DAT is lacking.

One of the basic issues confronting this research is determining where the breakdown of connected language in DAT occurs. Is it possible to transcend this descriptional level of "empty speech" and approach an explanation of narrative discourse deficit? Locating the origin or origins of such a narrative production deficit would shed light on the linguistic and general cognitive processes involved in the production of connected language.

Such an area of research is not without obstacles. Even a more constrained form of discourse than conversation, such as a monologic narrative in describing a picture, involves the integration of visuoperceptual information, ideas, concepts, schemas, communicative goals, and conceptual to linguistic mapping. The question of determining the relative contribution of each of these component processes in discourse as well as their interrelationships at first glance may appear overwhelmingly complex given the enormity of the behavioral function of discourse. Furthermore, there is no consensus among researchers on the critical components of narrative discourse since discourse analysis draws from a large field of models (e.g., de Beaugrande, 1980; Halliday & Hasan, 1976).

The "shotgun" approach, in which many arbitrarily different narrative tasks are administered along with a wealth of discourse measures, may be considered of limited value. The problem of specifying the loci of narrative deficit in the language of dementia should be amenable to experimental control by manipulating the characteristics of the narrative tasks. That is, systematically varying the conceptual and propositional structure of the narrative stimuli should permit a clearer view of where the breakdown in connected language occurs for the demented adult.

Ehrlich (1990) provided an example of this approach to the discourse deficits of DAT adults. The structure of narrative tasks was directly manipulated in order to control for the amount of content and picture format display. The relationship between narrative design and the narrative production allowed predictions about the suspected origins of deficit. The mode of picture display influenced neither the amount of content nor the grammatical performance for the DAT adults. In contrast, the amount of information pictorially represented significantly influenced the content produced by the DAT adults. My findings supported the contribution of both linguistic and broader cognitive systems to narrative discourse production.

Adding to our knowledge about the origins of deficit may also suggest therapeutic principles for professionals and paraprofessionals working with DAT patients and their families. Rehabilitation techniques frequently emerge from a clearer understanding of the disorder. One obvious example of clinical application is exploring the diagnostic and therapeutic usefulness of many of the discourse analysis techniques described.

Another important issue emerging from this body of research is the influence of the type of discourse task. As noted earlier, most of the studies lack sufficient experimental control of the form of discourse elicited. Although the amount and complexity of information to be conveyed in a narrative task is difficult to control, the content and format of the stimulus structure of the narrative requires such experimental manipulation. Further exploration of the effects of the design and presentation of such stimuli on the language production is necessary. Specifically, one might ask what relationship obtains between narrative structure and production for DAT adults; the interplay between dementia and narrative conditions might yield useful information about the nature of narrative breakdown. It is clear that the manipulation of format and presentation need to be studied further before its role on narrative production can be better specified.

Finally, implications for future research growing out of this literature on pathological narrative production can be addressed. Attention should be paid to methodological issues. This area of research would be enriched by continued refinement of discourse analysis. As discussed earlier, the techniques used for eliciting and analyzing discourse as well as the models for understanding discourse vary widely. Improvement in the measurement techniques applied to discourse analysis would permit better descriptions of the phenomena in question. Issues concerning discourse breakdown in DAT can only be studied if the tools that examine it operate with precision and sophistication. Additionally, models of normal narrative production would be better informed by more precise measurement techniques.

Improved discourse analysis techniques might allow other sorts of experimental manipulation of narrative tasks and stimuli. For example, experimental control of narrative schema, goals, and content might provide answers to the research questions. It might also prove useful to examine other possibly influential aspects of the narrative stimulus for DAT adults such as size of the stimuli and story structures. Perhaps, the addition of an orally presented narrative model would prove useful. Also, the effect of other types of visual stimuli (e.g., video) can be explored.

The broader question of determining where the breakdown of narrative production occurs in DAT adults is not likely to find a simple answer. Rather, it is probable that different directions of influence (e.g., semantic–lexical and ideational) merge to produce the pattern of narrative discourse associated with DAT. Multiple impairments to cognitive and linguistic subsystems are more likely responsible for the decrements in narrative production seen in DAT patients given the diffuse nature of the damage. It is also not clear how such ideational and semantic–lexical systems interact during narrative production. It is reasonable to expect that these two systems operate interdependently in connected language production. The unearthing of the interplay between cognitive and linguistic processes which underlie narrative production represents a long-term goal in neurolinguistic investigations of the language of DAT adults.

Another question to be addressed concerns the syntactic production of DAT adults. Because simplified syntax is evident in some studies, perhaps it is not as preserved in DAT as most researchers have suggested. Future studies should address production differences among various discourse genres. Additionally, future research should clarify the concept of tangentiality in discourse. An operational definition of this term would be a helpful first step. For example, it may prove useful to categorize as tangential all content items that remain after the target content is selected and scored.

Finally, two other directions for future research are offered here. Exploring the relationships of narrative production and semantic and episodic memories might add to our understanding of the nature of the impairment. Also, the pragmatics of narrative production should be further explored. There may be strategies for experimentally disentangling factors such as appreciating the listener's needs in connected language. Functional language measures applied to DAT adults may aim toward global assessment of communicative breakdown as well as revealing specific patterns of deficits.

The usefulness of research on demented discourse is well supported on both theoretical and clinical grounds. Any knowledge of the loci of narrative deficit may inform a model of normative discourse production and may shed light on the relationship between more narrowly defined linguistic processes and nonlinguistic cognitive capacities. Methodological and theoretical refinements should advance this area of research.

REFERENCES

Bayles, K. A. (1982). Language function in senile dementia. *Brain and Language, 16*, 265–280.

Bayles, K. A. (1986). Management of neurogenic communication disorders associated with dementia. In R. Chapey (Ed.), *Language intervention strategies in adult aphasia*. Baltimore, MD: Williams & Wilkins.

Bayles, K. A., & Boone, D. R. (1982). The potential of language tasks for identifying senile dementia. *Journal of Speech and Hearing Disorders, 47*, 210–217.

Bayles, K. A., & Kaszniak, A. W. (1987). *Communication and cognition in normal aging and dementia*. Boston, MA: College-Hill Press.

Beeson, P. M., Bayles, K. A., Tomoeda, C. K., & Slauson, T. J. (1987). *Oral discourse in demented, aphasic, and elderly individuals: Content analysis.* Paper presented at the annual meeting of the American Speech-Language Hearing Association, New Orleans, LA.

Davis, G. A., & Wilcox, M. J. (1985). *Adult aphasia rehabilitation.* San Diego, CA: College Hill Press.

de Beaugrande, R. (1980). Text, discourse, and process. Toward a multidisciplinary science of texts. In R. O. Freedle (Ed.), *Advances in discourse processes* (Vol. 4). Norwood, NJ: Ablex.

Ehrlich, J. (1990). *Influence of structure on the content of oral narrative in adults with dementia of the Alzheimer's type.* Unpublished doctoral dissertation, The City University of New York.

Goodglass, H., & Kaplan, E. (1983). *Boston diagnostic examination for aphasia.* Philadelphia: Lea & Febiger.

Halliday, M. A. K., & Hasan, R. (1976). *Cohesion in English.* London: Longman.

Hier, D. B., Hagenlocker, K., & Shindler, A. G. (1985). Language disintegration in dementia: Effects of etiology and severity. *Brain and Language, 25,* 117–133.

Horner, J., Heyman, A., Kanter, J., Royall, J. B., & Aker, C. R. (1983). *Longitudinal changes in spoken discourse in Alzheimer's démentia.* Paper presented at the annual meeting of the International Neuropsychological Society, Mexico City.

Irigaray, L. (1973). *Le langage des dements* [The language of dementia]. The Hague: Mouton.

Kempler, D., Curtiss, S., & Jackson, C. (1987). Syntactic preservation in Alzheimer's disease. *Journal of Speech and Hearing Research, 30,* 343–350.

Loban, W. (1976). *Language development: Kindergarten through grade 12* (*Res. Rep. No. 18*). Urbana, IL: National Council of Teachers of English.

Martin, A., & Fedio, P. (1983). Word production and comprehension in Alzheimer's disease: The breakdown of semantic knowledge. *Brain and Language, 19*(1), 124–141.

McKhann, G., Drachman, D., Folstein, M., Katzman, R., Price, D., & Stadlan, E. M. (1984). Clinical diagnosis of Alzheimer's disease: Report of the NINCDS-ADRDA Work Groups under the auspices of Dept. of Health and Human Services Task Force on Alzheimer's Disease. *Neurology, 34,* 939–944.

Nicholas, M., Obler, L. K., Albert, M. L., & Helm-Estabrooks, N. (1985). Empty speech in Alzheimer's disease and fluent aphasia. *Journal of Speech and Hearing Research, 28,* 405–410.

Obler, L. K. (1981). Review: Le Langage des déments, by Luce Irigary. *Brain and Language, 12,* 375–386.

Obler, L. K. (1983). Language and brain dysfunction in dementia. In S. Segalowitz (Ed.), *Language functions and brain organization.* New York: Academic Press.

Ripich, D. N., & Terrell, B. Y. (1988). Patterns of discourse cohesion and coherence in Alzheimer's disease. *Journal of Speech and Hearing Disorders, 53,* 8–15.

Santo Pietro, M. J., & Berman, R. (1984). *Analysis of connected speech in institutionalized elderly with and without senile dementia.* Paper presented at the annual meeting of the American Speech-Language Hearing Association, San Francisco, CA.

Schwartz, M., Marin, O., & Saffran, E. (1979). Dissociations of language function in dementia: A case study. *Brain and Language, 7,* 277–306.

Shekim, L. O., & LaPointe, L. L. (1984). *Production of discourse in individuals with Alzheimer's disease.* Paper presented at the 12th annual meeting of the International Neuropsychological Society, Houston, TX.

Smith, S. R., Chenery, H. J., & Murdoch, B. E. (1989). Semantic abilities in dementia of the Alzheimer's type. *Brain and Language, 36,* 533–542.

Ulatowska, H. K., Allard, L., Donnell, A., Bristow, J., Haynes, S., Flower, A., & North, A. J. (1988). Discourse performance in subjects with dementia of the Alzheimer's type. In H. A. Whitaker (Ed.), *Neuropsychological studies of non-focal brain damage.* New York: Springer-Verlag.

Ulatowska, H. K., & Bond, S. (1990). Discourse changes in dementia. In R. Lubinski (Ed.), *Dementia in communication: Research and clinical implications.* Philadelphia: B. C. Decker.

Ulatowska, H. K., Freedman-Stern, R., Weiss-Doyel, A., Macaluso-Haynes, S., & North, A. J. (1983). Production of narrative discourse in aphasia. *Brain and Language, 19*, 317–341.

Ulatowska, H. K., North, A. J., & Macaluso-Haynes, S. (1981). Production of narrative and procedural discourse in aphasia. *Brain and Language, 18*, 315–341.

Whitaker, H. A. (1976). A case of isolation of the language function. In H. Whitaker & H. A. Whitaker (Eds.), *Studies in neurolinguistics* (Vol. 2, pp.). New York: Academic Press.

Yorkston, E., & Beukelman, D. (1980). An analysis of connected speech samples of aphasic and normal speakers. *Journal of Speech and Hearing Disorders, 45*, 27–36.

Chapter 10

Conversational Topic-Shifting Analysis in Dementia

Linda J. Garcia
University of Ottawa and Ottawa General Hospital

Yves Joanette
Centre de Recherche du Centre Hospitalier Côte-des-Neiges and University of Montreal

Speech–language pathologists are increasingly called upon to differentially diagnose aphasia and language of dementia. Although traditional aphasia tests may give some insight into the language deficit in dementia, such an impairment is not always well understood. Yet the experienced speech–language pathologist will subjectively identify the conversational discourse of the dementia patient as somewhat unusual or incoherent in comparison to the aphasic. Few available standard aphasia batteries can identify the subtle differences between aphasia and the language of dementia often noted by the experienced clinician.

In order to better understand the nature of the differences between aphasic discourse and discourse in dementia and of those between normal and disordered discourse, it is important to develop adequate descriptive tools. After reviewing the literature on conversational discourse and dementia, this chapter addresses some of the concepts that need to be considered when attempting to develop such tools. Comments are made regarding the importance of identifying whether the problem at hand is a sequential one (i.e., relating to the links between sequential units of conversation) or an interpretive one (i.e., relating to the underlying interpretation of the conversation unit). The rationale for using a text-processing model and for addressing the issue of relevance is discussed. Using this information as a theoretical framework, a study looking at conversational discourse in dementia is used to illustrate some of the patterns that can be observed in incoherent conversations. Results are then explained in terms of a text processing theoretical model.

CONVERSATIONAL DISCOURSE AND DEMENTIA

Conversational discourse in dementia has not enjoyed an outpouring of systematic research. Initially, most published papers related anecdotal comments. Irigaray (1967) described demented patients as being "incoherent" with an absence of "real control" over their utterances. De Ajuriaguerra and Tissot (1975) noted that terms implicit in the situation were omitted. Ernst, Dalby, and Dalby (1970) noted a "lack of language initiative." Obler (1979) and Obler and Albert (1981) found patients with dementia to have little communicative intent and to repeat material more often.

The increased attention linguists have given to discourse analysis has encouraged investigators to go beyond the anecdotal observations and into a more systematic analysis of these patients' communicative abilities. In her doctoral dissertation, Campbell-Taylor (1984) looked at what professionals and nonprofessionals identified as being unusual in the conversations of a dementia of the Alzheimer's type (DAT) patient and an examiner. The more prominent categories selected by both groups reflected a pragmatic deficit. Dementing patients were found to make inappropriate topic shifts, have disordered eye gaze, and abnormal content in their conversations. Ripich, Terrell, and Spinelli (1983) found their dementia patient to use structural cohesive ties but the semantics of the discourse was unrelated. In a later study, Ripich and Terrell (1988) looked at cohesion and coherence during topic-directed interviews using subjects with DAT and normal elderly subjects. Results showed that DAT patients used more than twice as many words and more than four times as many turns as the normal controls. DAT subjects were less impaired in their structural cohesion than in what the authors called *semantic cohesion.* Absence of a referent was the most frequent *cohesive* error in DAT. Information errors were the most frequent type of errors associated with *incoherence.* Interestingly, the interviewers also altered their conversational discourse to suit their conversational partner. They produced more words and turns with the DAT subjects than when speaking to the normal elderly.

Illes (1986, 1989) also looked at the conversational skills of patients with dementia. Her subjects were interviewed and asked to respond to questions about various personal topics. Illes found the patterns of spontaneous language in patients with Alzheimer's disease, Huntington's disease, and Parkinson's disease to be significantly different from each other and from the language in her normal elderly subjects. She found that unlike DAT patients, Parkinson's disease and Huntington's disease patients had a "press of speech." In addition, Huntington's disease patients differed from normals in their syntactic complexity but not so for the Parkinson's disease patients. She found a significant increase in the number of long silent hesitations, a significant increase in the number of self-corrections, and a significant increase in the number of aborted phrases in patients with Alzheimer's disease.

Hutchinson and Jensen (1980) compared five dementing elderly females to five normal elderly females in a nursing home for an evaluation of their conversational discourse skills. They found the dementing individuals to have more turns and fewer utterances per turn, which suggested that they did not elaborate on their topic. The experimental group also made extensive presuppositions regarding shared knowledge. They initiated new topics more and violated rules of continuation of one's own topic and partner's topic.

The process of deterioration of pragmatic skills in dementia is not well understood. Ripich, Vertes, Whitehouse, and Fulton (1988) attempted to determine some of the processes involved in DAT conversations. Their study involved 11 normal elderly and 11 DAT subjects in a 9-minute unstructured conversation that had been disguised as a coffee break from regular clinic testing. Conversations between the examiner and either a DAT subject or a normal elderly subject were transcribed and analyzed according to Dore's (1975, 1979) classification of speech acts. Results showed that the normal elderly used more words per turn, more assertions, and made more responses to choice questions. The DAT subjects used more process questions ("why" and "how" questions). The examiner made more requests with the normal elderly, asked more process questions, and used more descriptions. The examiner used more words per turn, more action requests, and asked more clarification questions when speaking with the DAT subjects.

In reviewing the scant literature on conversational discourse of subjects with DAT, one apparent difficulty is the absence of an explicit theoretical framework. This deficiency makes it difficult to make comparisons among studies. It is also probably responsible for the somewhat general nature of the descriptions reported. One reason for this may be that conceptual frameworks for conversational discourse have only been available recently. Moreover, the precise choice for a given conceptual framework is complicated by the fact that many different and sometimes opposing views abound in that field. Two theoretical concepts that impact the analysis of conversations in DAT are reviewed here. The first concept deals with the contrasting issues of sequencing and interpretation. The second deals with the concept of relevance.

INTERPRETIVE VERSUS SEQUENTIAL ISSUES

Two problems are raised by the analysis of conversational discourse, according to Moeschler (1993). The first is a *sequencing problem* "which consists in explaining the connections between utterance units in conversation, and more specifically the connections marked by discourse or pragmatic connectives" (p. 149). The second is an *interpretive problem*, which "consists in explaining the relation between an utterance-type and its interpretation" (p. 149). In the first sense, the researcher is interested in how the utterances are "connected" to previous and following utterances from an organizational, structural standpoint. In the second sense, the researcher is interested in the underlying propositional meaning relationships. In order to develop useful tools for the analysis of conversation in clinical populations, the researcher/clinician needs to identify whether the analysis will address the issue of utterance sequencing or the issue of utterance interpretation .

In the case of DAT, much of the literature on conversational discourse points to a problem with pragmatics in these patients. The question remains as to whether a pragmatic problem reflects an interpretive or a sequential issue. If pragmatics is seen as concerned with the identification of the illocutionary force or the underlying, intended meaning, then it is clearly an interpretive issue. If a pragmatic problem is seen as a difficulty with the use of language in its broadest sense, then it could be a sequential issue. In this latter interpretation, the researcher wishes to address the manner in which DAT patients place their utterances in the overall sequential organization of the conversation. In the former interpretation, the researcher wishes to address the manner in which DAT patients "translate" their intended meanings into utterances and how these meanings are interconnected in the conversation. Because it does not address structural issues of conversation, investigation into an interpretive problem can be motivated by a theory of discourse processing that does not address conversational discourse per se. In contrast, investigation into a sequential problem must be motivated by a theory of action such as speech act theory (Austin, 1962; Searle, 1965, 1969, 1975). In Moeschler's (1993) viewpoint, "the sequencing problem, which is specific to discourse, is neither a linguistic nor a pragmatic problem, but depends on a theory of action; on the other hand, the interpretive problem is not specific to conversation, and is better described in a framework which is independent of conversational data" (p. 154).

The majority of studies thus far on conversational discourse in dementia point to a problem with pragmatic issues relating to underlying meaning. This type of problem can be manifested, for instance, by a difficulty in maintaining topic. In Moeschler's terms this would address an interpretive problem. Therefore, investigation into the topic maintenance question in DAT need not rely on a theory of action such as speech act theory but can rely on a theory of discourse processing. In addition, theoretical considerations of issues of relevance, although not concerned with conversational discourse per se, may help explain why DAT patients have incoherent discourse.

THE CONCEPT OF RELEVANCE

In conversation, it is, at least initially, the theme or topic of the conversation that constitutes the unifying factor (Goldberg, 1983). In making a relevant contribution to conversation, a speaker must realize at least two important steps: (a) identify the main point or topic (a receptive process), and (b) produce an utterance that is connected semantically to the hearer's interpretation of this topic (an expressive process).

In understanding a speaker, the hearer tries to determine how the speaker's utterances relate to the main point in the conversation, to information stored in memory about the speaker, previous interactions, shared knowledge, and to information in the immediate environment. The hearer then redefines what the topic of conversation is, based on these global conclusions (Wardhaugh, 1985) and makes judgments of relevance and coherency as the conversation evolves (Goldberg, 1983; Tracy & Moran, 1983). In determining relevance, having a notion of topic is crucial to making a pertinent contribution (McLaughlin, 1984).

In text-processing terms, the identification of a topic or gist is, in essence, the formulation of a macrostructure and identification of a macroproposition (see Kintsch, 1988; Kintsch & Van Dijk, 1978; Van Dijk, 1977, 1980, 1981; Van Dijk & Kintsch, 1983). The formulation of this macrostructure is done using a variety of strategies. According to this theory, incoming information can be deleted or amalgamated with information stored in memory in order to arrive at the main point. Should there be some missing propositional information, the reader (in text-processing terms) or the hearer (in conversation-processing terms) makes inferences and supplements missing information based on information found in memory. In conversational discourse, this process becomes complex because macroprocessing must be done on-line and must include a multitude of topic shifts. The hearer (no longer the reader) must process the information as it is presented. There is no chance to return to previously presented material as in a written text. Forming an idea of the gist or macrostructure must clearly be done on-line.

As this macrostructure is being formulated, the speaker plans an utterance that will hopefully be relevant to the conversation. In order to make a relevant contribution, the speaker must try to relate the expressed proposition to the set of propositions in the hearer's accessible memory (Wilson & Sperber, 1981). Based on the identification of the previous macrostructure, the speaker will give as much information as necessary for the hearer to identify the new macroproposition. The amount of information that is shared with the hearer is dependent on the same pragmatic information necessary for interpretation. That is, the speaker will consider what is known about the hearer, previous interactions, and so forth.

Whether or not an item is actually considered "relevant" is ultimately determined by the interpreter. It is up to the hearer to "infer or invent a situationally plausible, topically relevant motive for the communicator's having included the item" (Sanders, 1983, p. 69). Thus, relevance is not a categorical entity but rather a matter of degree (Tracy, 1982). This theory of relevance stresses that the hearer, when faced with the propositions given by the speaker, will process them in relation to propositions already held in his or her own memory and in relation to a whole gamut of pragmatic information.

Conversational partners must continuously adjust their information-processing skills from role of speaker to role of hearer and vice versa. As speakers they must make contributions that will be relevant to their own interpretation of the macroproposition based on the strategies for macroprocessing and based on information stored in their memories. As hearers they must make sense of what is presented to them on-line by the speaker by forming a new macroproposition and relating it to information in memory, thereby attaching relevance to the speaker's utterance. The complexity of this process is overwhelming if one considers the array of topic shifts that occur in conversation. Likewise, if one must hold propositions in memory in order to process further incoming propositions, it is evident that patients with a known working memory deficit would have difficulty maintaining a relevant conversation.

In conclusion, several points can be retained. First, if in fact DAT patients have difficulty maintaining a coherent conversation, this may be due to a difficulty in manipulating topic. In order to manipulate topic, one needs to have some form of interpretation of what that topic is—hence, it becomes an interpretive issue in Moeschler's terms. Second, assuming it is an interpretive issue, one does not need to rely on speech act theory to help explain the phenomenon observed. A text-processing model that is independent of conversational data, such as the one proposed by Kintsch and Van Dijk, can be a satisfactory choice. This theory gives the investigator a theoretical framework from which to explain how information can be structured to form an idea of topic (or macrostructure). Third, in order to maintain a coherent conversation, one must be relevant. Relevance is determined by the hearer as he or she determines the relationship between the speaker's proposition and the propositional information in his or her own memory.

The following study is an example of how one can operationalize the description of an interpretive problem (i.e., topic shifting) in the analysis of the conversational discourse of demented and normal elderly subjects. Because relevance is of the utmost importance in the conversational discourse of DAT patients, utterances are analyzed with regards to their relevance to the topic of conversation. More precisely, this study aims at describing, as specifically as possible, the topic-shifting profiles of patients with DAT in comparison to those found in normal elderly subjects. In attempting to clarify the interpretive problem, the study explores the basic structure of topic manipulation (e.g., percentage of topic maintenance and topic shifts; place of shift), the technique used to shift the topic, the possible reasons for the occurrence of the shift, and the contexts to which the shift occurred, including the role of knowledge.

METHODOLOGY

Subjects

There were 10 subjects, 4[1] with probable DAT following the NINCDS-ADRDA work group criteria (McKhann et al., 1984), 5 normal elderly (NE), and 1 normal

[1]There were originally five subjects tested in this study. One of these subjects (Subject A1) had her diagnosis reconsidered at her 6-month follow-up visit. Her diagnosis was changed from DAT to multi-infarct dementia. For this reason, she and her partner are excluded from the graphs presented here. Her results are, however, interesting for demonstration purposes. They are briefly discussed toward the end of this chapter.

middle-aged adult (S.W.), who served as conversational partner for all subjects. All subjects were female, over age 65 (except S.W.), high school educated (except one), and monolingual English speakers. Almost all subjects were Canadian born with Canadian-born parents thereby coming from the same cultural background (Table 10.1). All had adequate hearing for one-to-one conversation as determined by audiological examination.

In addition to receiving the necessary neuropsychological and medical tests for diagnosis, all DAT subjects received a full Boston Diagnostic Aphasia Examination (Goodglass & Kaplan, 1976) and had a Global Deterioration Scale rating of 5 (Reisberg, Ferris, De Leon, & Crook, 1982). In order to eliminate the effects of institutionalization (Lubinski, 1984) on subjects' conversational skills, all DAT subjects were living in their own homes at time of testing.

Each normal healthy elderly subject was matched for age and education to a single DAT subject. The conversational partner for all subjects was 42 years of age and a professional social worker who was familiar with DAT patients but not with these particular subjects.

TABLE 10.1
Subject Demographic Information

Subject	*Sex*	*Age*	*Education*	*Past Occupation*	*Subject's Place of Birth*	*Parent's Place of Birth*
A2 (DAT)	Fem.	69	Grade 8	housewife	Ottawa	Quebec (F) Ontario (M)
N2 (NE)	Fem.	67	secondary	secretary	Ottawa	England (F) Ottawa (M)
A3 (DAT)	Fem.	73	secondary	clerical/ sales	St. John, N.B.	Nova Scotia (F), New Brunswick (M)
N3 (NE)	Fem.	74	Grade 10, commercial	secretary	Ottawa	Ottawa (F) England (M)
A4 (DAT)	Fem.	72	secondary	secretary	Fredericton	New Brunswick (both F and M)
N4 (NE)	Fem.	71	secondary	secretary	England; moved at 2.5 years of age.	Ireland (F) England (M)
A5 (DAT)	Fem.	74	secondary	housewife	Carleton Place, Ontario	Carleton Place, Ontario (both F and M)
N5 (NE)	Fem.	72	secondary	housewife	Ottawa	Ottawa (both F and M)

Note. DAT = Dementia of the Alzheimer type, NE = normal elderly, Fem. = female, F = father's place of birth, M = mother's place of birth.

Procedure

All subjects were videotaped in their own homes using a Sony Handicam video 8 camera Model no. CCD-F40 fitted on a tripod. In addition, the conversation was recorded on a Sony two-channel cassette recorder Model No. TC-D5M using two Sony F-25 table-top microphones. Subjects were asked to converse about any topic they desired for 1 hour. All conversations were between the subject and the social worker, S.W. In order to allow for proper analysis of subjects' skills in topic shifting, there were no restrictions on the topics discussed. Because the interest was in topic-shifting behavior, it was important that topic initiating not be biased toward the social worker as in a topic-directed interview—this would have been self-defeating. Restricting what is said in a conversation is counterproductive to studying face-to-face interactions (Holtgraves, Srull, & Socall, 1989; Levinson, 1983; Murphy, 1990). For this reason, neither the subjects nor the social worker were aware of the specific goal of the study.

Transcriptions of the conversations were made for each subject–social worker pair. The first and last 15 minutes of the hour-long conversation were omitted from transcription in order to minimize any possible initial effects of video recording and to eliminate the openings/closings of the conversations. A speaker's turn ceased the moment the other conversational partner began to speak.

Transcripts were reviewed with the videotape, in order to insert any descriptive comments where necessary. For example, comments included occurrences in the environment (e.g., a telephone ringing), or impressions of the speaker's intention (e.g., "Uhm-uhm" meaning "yes" vs. "Uhm-uhm" used as conversational support). Interpretation of these was made based on supralinguistic/nonverbal information (e.g., facial expression, intonation). Turns were numbered in sequence and the speaker was identified by her initials.

Categorization

Each turn was evaluated in terms of its relation to the topic. A *topic* was defined as the macroproposition of the exchange as interpreted by the analyzers. The major unit of analysis was the *topic unit*, defined as a set of continuous utterances appearing to relate to the same topic without being separated by introduction or renewal of another topic or of a shift in turn. Topic units were first categorized globally as either a topic maintenance, a topic shift, or "undetermined." All those falling into the topic-shift category were further classified into each of the categories of place of shift, the type of shift, the possible reasons for the shift, and the context to which the shift might have related. Within each of these more general categories, each topic-shift unit was codified into one of the subcategories (e.g., topic initiation, see Table 10.2). The first author and two other speech–language pathologists arrived at a consensus in the categorization of topic units. Operational definitions of these categories are given in the appendix.

TABLE 10.2
Topic Shift Categories

Category	*Subcategories*
Global	Topic maintenance
	Semantic
	Nonsemantic
	Topic shift
	Undetermined
Topic Shifts Only	
Place of shift	Within turn (WT)
	Across turn (AT)
Type of shift	Topic initiation (TI)
	Topic shading (TS)
	Renewal (R)
	Insert (I)
	Unexpected (UT)
	Undetermined (UD)
Reason for shift	End of topic (ET)
	Decreased comprehension (DC)
	Fail to continue (FC)
	Outside stimulus (OS)
	Repetition of idea (RI)
	Anecdotal (A)
	Unknown (U)
Context	Text (T)
	Environment (E)
	Specific knowledge (SK)
	General knowledge (GK)
	Unknown (U)

All categorizations were later stored in a computerized database (Revelation Technologies, 1987) and from these data, a general and subject profile could be extracted. The general profile was expressed as (a) a percentage of all productions in the conversations, including both conversers, and (b) each converser's contribution to the conversation. Its aim was to give a global graphic representation of the conversation. Number of shifts, maintenances (both semantic and nonsemantic), and undetermined were calculated as a percentage of the total number of turns in the conversation. Categories within place, type, reason, and context were calculated as a percentage of the total number of topic shifts in the conversation.

The subject profile was expressed as a percentage of each subject's productions, excluding those made by the other conversational partner. Number of shifts, maintenances (both semantic and nonsemantic), and undetermined were calculated as a percentage of the total number of *turns produced by that speaker* (i.e., DAT or NE) in the conversation. Categories within place, type, reason, and context were calculated as a percentage of the total number of topic *shifts produced by that speaker* (i.e., DAT or NE) in the conversation.

RESULTS

The present study did not use a group design, thus only large differences could be considered of any interest and these are often best examined through visual analysis (Hegde, 1987; McReynolds & Kearns, 1983). Data representing some of the more salient results are presented for the purpose of illustrating the patterns that can be observed, and for providing data that can illustrate some of the analytic discourse concepts discussed. Following a description of the graphic data, the results are discussed in relation to the theoretical framework presented in this chapter. The chapter concludes with some reflection as to the applicability of this methodology. A more complete description of this data and other results not presented here is available elsewhere (Garcia & Joanette, 1994).

Type of Shift: Topic Shading

Operational Definition. *Topic shading* "introduces a new topic by first establishing its relevance to or connection with the topic that has been on the floor" (Crow, 1983, pp. 142). Establishing its relevance could be done through repetition of a referent, pronominal referencing or using connecting phrases like "Speaking of. . . ."

Topic shading requires that the converser hold the previous topic in memory and relate the new topic to the old one. It assumes the ability to be coherent. Considering the documented memory difficulties of DAT subjects and the theories postulated regarding the use of memory in discourse, one might expect DAT subjects to have proportionately lower percentages of topic-shading shifts.

This pattern was obvious in three of the four pairs of conversations (Fig. 10.1). The topic shading that did exist in the DAT conversations was mostly S.W.'s (Fig. 10.2). Subject A4 was the only subject who did not show this pattern, having as equal an amount of topic shading as S.W.

Reason for Shift: Failure to Continue

Operational Definition. *Failure to continue* describes a situation in which a member of the dyad decides or is unable to continue an ongoing unfinished topic, thereby forcing the other member of the dyad to change the topic because of a lack of continuity.

Research findings indicating that DAT subjects do not elaborate on their topic and have more aborted phrases, allow one to speculate that there would be an increased proportion of these shifts in the DAT conversations. One could also

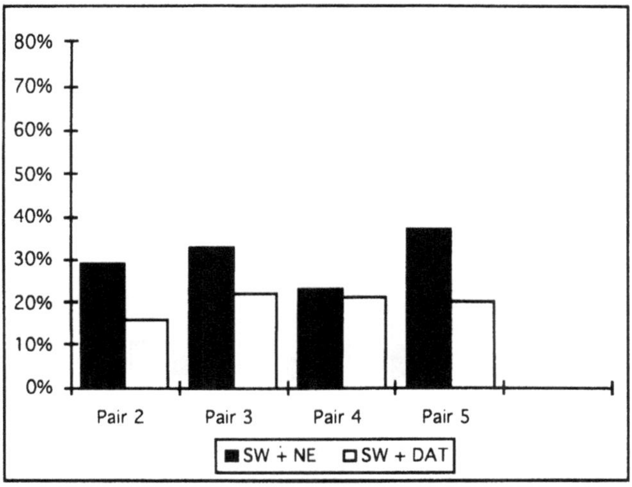

FIG. 10.1. General profile: Topic shading. Percentage of *topic shading* shifts in the total number of topic shifts in the conversation for both NE/S.W. conversations (S.W.+NE) and DAT/S.W. conversations (S.W.+DAT).

speculate that the majority of these shifts would be due to S.W. If the DAT subject cannot continue her topic, S.W. would be in a position to change topics because of this lack of continuation.

Figure 10.3 supported this expectation. All pairs of conversations showed a proportionately larger percentage of shifts for this reason in the DAT conversations, with the majority of these being due to S.W. (Fig. 10.4).

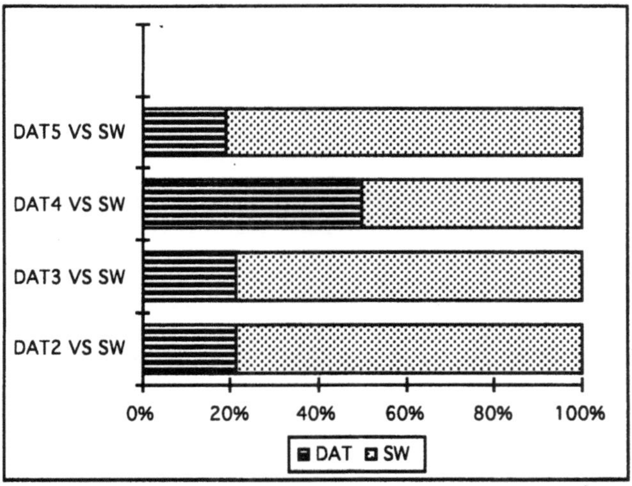

FIG. 10.2. Contribution: Topic shading. Relative contribution of each conversational partner to the total percentage of *topic shading* shifts for DAT/S.W. conversations (S.W.+DAT).

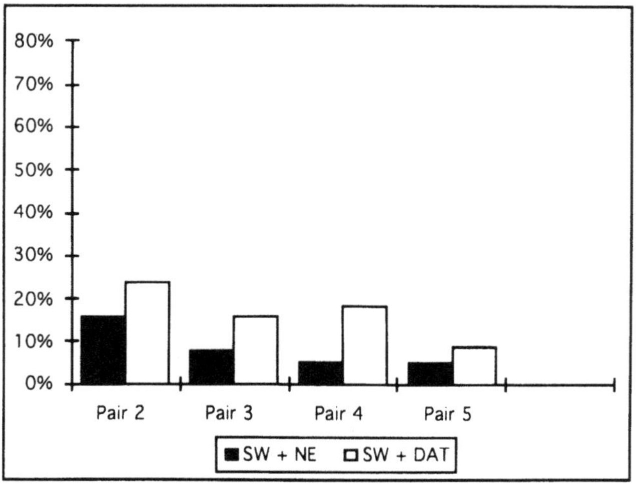

FIG. 10.3. General profile: Failure to continue. Percentage of shifts due to *failure to continue* in the total number of topic shifts in the conversation for both NE/S.W. conversations (S.W.+NE) and DAT/S.W. conversations (S.W.+DAT).

Reason for Shift: Anecdotal

Operational Definition. An *anecdotal shift* is a topic shift that has occurred because of a desire to share a short story, usually biographical in nature.

Anecdotes may be considered little topics tangential to the previous topic or illustrations of a previous topic. In order to illustrate a point with a small

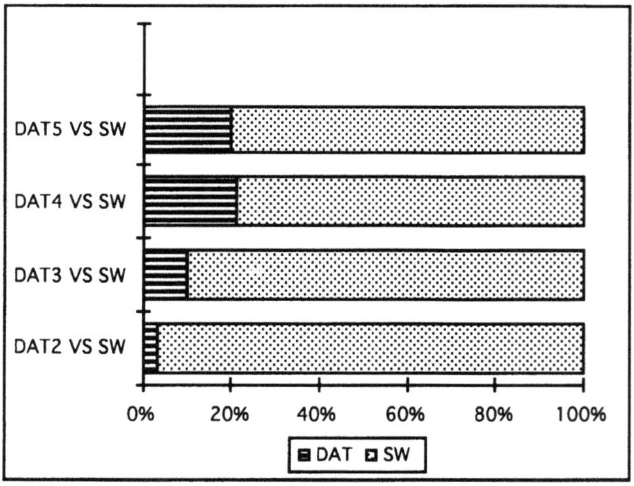

FIG. 10.4. Contribution: Failure to continue. Relative contribution of each conversational partner to the total percentage of shifts due to *failure to continue* for DAT/S.W. conversations (S.W.+DAT).

autobiographical story, one needs to be able to identify the main topic (i.e., the macrostructure) and keep it in memory so that the anecdote is relevant. In light of this, one may suspect that there would be a larger proportion of anecdotal shifts in conversations with NE subjects because one might assume that their memories are capable of holding the information in memory.

Examination of Fig. 10.5 supported this premise in all cases. This was again reflected in terms of individual analyses of the subjects' profiles (Fig. 10.6). The NE subjects were proportionately more likely than the DAT subjects to shift a topic because of a desire to tell an anecdote.

DISCUSSION

One of the basic premises of the Kintsch and Van Dijk (1978) theory as presented in this chapter is that propositional information is processed in cycles using a series of strategies that enable the hearer to attach the incoming information to information stored in secondary memories. This enables the hearer to form a macrostructure and arrive at a macroproposition that is, in essence, a topic.

Even in this schematic representation of a very complex model, it is obvious that it presupposes the proper functioning of many linguistic and psychological functions unavailable to the neurologically impaired subject. In the case of DAT, impairment of working and/or semantic and/or episodic and/or explicit–implicit memories would clearly affect the ability to build a macrostructure. When information is presented orally as in conversation, macroprocessing is done

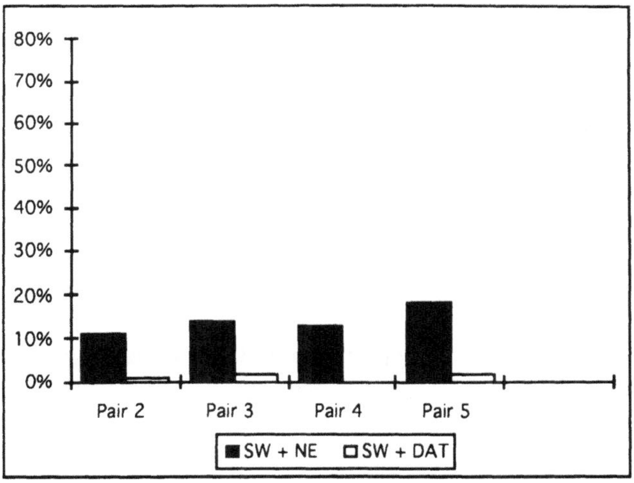

FIG. 10.5. General profile: Anecdotes. Percentage of shifts due to *anecdotes* in the total number of topic shifts in the conversation for both NE/S.W. conversations (S.W.+NE) and DAT/S.W. conversations (S.W.+DAT).

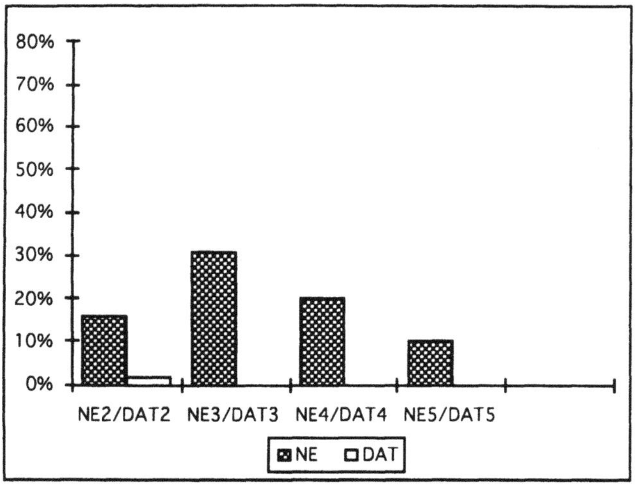

FIG. 10.6. Subject profile: Anecdotes. Percentage of shifts due to *anecdotes* in the total number of topic shifts produced by each individual subject (NE or DAT), irrespective of the conversational partner, S.W.

on-line (Lorch, Lorch, & Matthews, 1985) and uses all kinds of pragmatic information (Van Dijk, 1977). Hence, the demands on memory of macroprocessing in conversational discourse may be greater. Propositions need to be retained, deleted, reconstructed, or amalgamated with other information in the hearer's accessible memory as it is presented by the conversational partner.

In the following paragraphs, the results presented in this chapter are explained with a text-processing model as theoretical framework.

> Result 1: There were proportionately more topic shadings in the conversations with the NE subjects.

Explanation of Result 1 requires consideration of the notion of *topic shading*. Topic shading demands a certain conversational "finesse." Although Brinton and Fujiki (1984) analyzed discourse in children, the examiners in the present investigation had similar difficulties determining exactly where in the discourse the topic was shaded. This difficulty suggested that the shift of topic was done with a certain amount of skill on the part of the speaker. Brinton and Fujiki pointed out that the conversers appeared to be using this strategy in order to shift a topic while maintaining the overall coherence in the discourse.

Topic shading may signal that speakers are aware of the maxims of conversation and have chosen to simply notify their partners that they will violate the maxim of relevance (Grice, 1975). They make this transition easier for the listeners by providing the information necessary to link the present macroproposition to previously stated ones. This might mean that the speaker is not entrusting the listener with the task of selecting the appropriate propositions to store in the working memory buffer to await further processing (Kintsch & Van Dijk, 1978). When processing in cycles, a speaker, not allowing the listener the task of choosing appropriate propositions, will "begin each new sentence by repeating a crucial phrase from the old one" (p. 368). Topic shading is more than just repeating a phrase from previous propositions but the concept presented here might be generalized to topic-shifting skills. By definition *topic shading* explicitly relates the present, new topic to the old one. Hypothetically, DAT subjects (a) may not be aware that they should signal any violations of the maxim of relevance, and/or (b) may not have enough discursive skill to facilitate transition from one topic to the next.

> Result 2: There were proportionately more shifts as a result of a failure to continue the topic in conversations with the DAT subjects and the majority of these were due to S.W.

Result 2 agrees with the literature that suggests that DAT subjects have problems elaborating on a topic of conversation. If the DAT subjects did not elaborate on their topics or those of their partner's, S.W. would be forced to change the topic to keep the conversation flowing. In text-processing terms, the DAT subjects' memories might not allow them to form a macrostructure quickly enough with the incoming propositional information. Hence, it might be difficult for them to identify the macroproposition (or topic) and subsequently elaborate on its contents.

> Result 3: There were proportionately more shifts because of a desire to tell an anecdote in the conversations with the NE subjects.

Shifting a topic because of a desire to share an anecdote might be considered as a desire to shift in order to digress. However, such shifting demands that the conversational partner hold the previous information in temporary relevance while the *anecdote* is being shared. Unlike the problem discussed with the previous result (i.e., difficulty in identifying the macroproposition), this result might suggest a difficulty with the retention of such a macroproposition during the formation of a second macrostructure. In other words, the DAT subject must first identify Macroproposition 1, which is the topic prior to the anecdote. He or she must hold this topic in "marginal" relevance in memory because there is no evidence in the conversation (based on pragmatic information) that the topic has ended. While the subject is holding this topic in marginal relevance, he or she must process the new, incoming propositions that will make up Macroproposition 2, which will be the topic of the anecdote. This is theoretically impossible with an impaired memory system. In fact, it is likely impossible or nearly impossible with other impaired cognitive functions such as attention.

Applicability of the Methodology

The present study was offered as an example of how one might operationalize the analysis of an interpretive problem (i.e., topic shifting) in conversational discourse. It also aimed to offer an alternative to using speech act theory as a theoretical framework to the analysis of conversation. The following section critically evaluates the applicability of this methodology and its usefulness in both research and clinical applications.

As a research tool, the methodology proves to have several restrictions. First, as with other methods used for the analysis of natural conversations, this type of methodology is not open to group design or to systematic control of output. Because it aims to look at topic-shifting behavior, this type of analysis cannot have the amount of control that even a topic-directed interview may have. As a consequence, analyses remain subjective. Second, there is some doubt regarding the usefulness of the *global dimension* categories (i.e., percentage of shifts, maintenance—both semantic and nonsemantic—and undetermined) and the *place of shift* (i.e., within, across turn) categories as they were defined in this study. Third, the analysis of data in a consensus fashion should be reexamined. It was hypothesized at the outset that the novelty and subjectivity of such a classificatory system would lead to insurmountable problems in analyzing the data. It was also thought that the experimenter's assistance was necessary to explain the context in which the conversational items were shared, because the experimenter was present for all conversations. Thus, a consensus among three speech–language pathologists was judged as the most appropriate methodology. In reality, the categorization was quickly learned by the speech–language pathologists and any problems in the comprehension of context was readily available from the videotape. In subsequent studies, one may strongly consider an interjudge reliability component to the analysis, thereby making the results more robust.

This being said, the present methodology offers some interesting new avenues. First, it truly addresses one of the major interpretive problems of conversational discourse in DAT (i.e., the inability to maintain topic). Second, unlike previous studies that may try to describe the conversational discourse in its entirety, this methodology focuses on only one facet of natural conversation. Third, it encourages and gives a rationale for using theoretical models other than speech act theory. Finally, the methodology is able to pick up differences between subjects although it has not yet shown any reliability for making differential diagnoses. One of the more dramatic sets of results showing differences among subjects are those of Subject A1.

A1's data was not presented here (see footnote 1) because she does not present with DAT, although this was not known at the time of the study. Her present working diagnosis is multi-infarct dementia. Although she had not originally been chosen as a dissimilar subject, her topic-shifting profile was often very different from the other four DAT subjects.

In several instances, her profile resembled that of a normal subject's rather than that of a DAT subject's profile. In terms of the shifts due to failure to continue, the conversation with A1 had proportionately fewer than even her matched NE subject. Although there were proportionately fewer inserts and shifts for anecdotal reasons in the DAT subject; A1 was not obviously different from the normals in both these cases. Finally, S.W. did the majority of topic initiations with the DAT subjects. This was not the case with A1. The methodology and/or the raters were able to tease out a different topic-shifting profile in a subject who turned out to be different from the others, all the while assuming that this subject was no different from the other four. The reasons for these differences, of course, could not be explained objectively using this design. It could be that different etiologies give different discourse profiles, it could be that A1 was less severely impaired than the DAT subjects or it could reflect normal interindividual variation (see Obler et al., chapter 2, this volume). Nonetheless, a different pattern was identified using this methodology.

As a clinical tool, the methodology has the same restrictions just mentioned. In addition to the same advantages the tool may have for research, the methodology is conducive to studying partner influence or adaptation to incoherent discourse. For example, the clinician may be interested in seeing how family members help in keeping a conversation on topic. The methodology could also be applied to other clinical populations but the subcategories may prove to be very different across clinical groups.

CONCLUSIONS

This study presents a feasible means of describing one facet of natural conversation despite certain limitations. The methods used for this description were motivated in part by pragmatic and discourse-processing concepts. These theoretical notions served as a basis for interpreting and quantifying abstract concepts such as *relevance* and *coherence*, which were reported in the literature as being a major area of difficulty for adults with dementia. Based on prior reports in the literature, it was concluded that meaning relationships in these discourses may be best described through a detailed analysis of topic-shifting behavior.

Literature on brain-damaged subjects referred to "appropriate" and "inappropriate" topic shifting, yet what is appropriate or inappropriate was rarely defined. The human communication research literature reveals a body of knowledge regarding topic shifting that has only minimally been integrated into research focusing on brain-damaged populations. The present study illustrates some applications of this knowledge and stresses the need for further investigation of topic-shifting behavior. Being faced with the challenge of describing the nature of this *interpretive problem*, it was insufficient to rely on a speech act theory model alone.

APPENDIX: OPERATIONAL DEFINITIONS

1. Global Categories

Topic Maintenance

> Acts that maintain or terminate an established topic. . . . Once a topic has the floor, all acts that fall within the range of the conversation occupied by that topic may be coded as contributing to the maintenance of the topic. (Crow, 1983, pp. 140–141)

Maintenance of topic was not categorized in detail because it was not the focus of this research, aside from giving a global dimension. A distinction was made between those maintenances that contributed semantic information and those that did not. A *topic unit* judged to repeat or add some semantic information to the conversation was called a *semantic* Topic Maintenance. A *topic unit* judged as not contributing any semantic information to the conversation (e.g., "Uhm-uhm") was called a *nonsemantic* Topic Maintenance. This latter category was used mostly as conversational supports and were similar to what Goodenough and Weiner (1978) referred to as *passing moves*.

Aside from topic *maintenance*, a *topic unit* could be judged as a topic shift or *undetermined*. A topic unit judged as not continuing the immediately preceding identified topic was considered a *topic shift*. Third, if it was uncertain whether a topic unit maintained or shifted the previous topic, the unit was identified as *undetermined*.

2. Topic Shift Categories

Further classification was done on topic shifts only. The following classificatory system was primarily modeled on Crow (1983) with information extracted from Keenan and Schieffelin (1976), Planalp and Tracy (1980), and Van Dijk (1977). Each topic shift was coded for place, type, reason for shift, and the context to which it related.

1. Place of Shift

1.1. Within Turn. Within turn is a topic shift that occurred in the same turn as the preceding topic.

1.2. Across Turn. This is a topic shift that occurred across the turn boundaries.

2. Type of Shift

2.1. Topic Initiation. Topic initiation is "an attempt to introduce a new topic either at the beginning of a conversation, after a prior topic has been apparently terminated or after a period of nontopical talk ("drift") or silence" (Crow, 1983, p. 141).

2.2. Topic Shading. Topic shading "introduces a new topic by first establishing its relevance to or connection with the topic that has been on the floor" (Crow, 1983, p. 142). Establishing its relevance could be done through repetition of a referent, pronominal referencing, or using connecting phrases like "Speaking of. . . ."

2.3. Renewal. Renewal is "a shift back to an earlier topic after one or more other topics or topic-shifting attempts have intervened" (Crow, 1983, p. 144). These may or may not be marked (e.g., "Getting back to . . .").

2.4. Insert. Crow defined an *insert* as "An (often) abrupt shift that does not succeed in gaining the topical floor" (p. 148). These most often occurred within a turn. The shift was often tangential to the earlier topic but not marked as in topic shading. In an insert the impression was that the speakers did not want to drop the last topic discussed.

2.5. Unexpected. "An abrupt shift that succeeds in gaining the topical floor" is the definition Crow (1983, p. 146) gave for *unexpected.* These might have occurred during an unexpected occurrence in the environment (e.g., a telephone ringing).

2.6. Undetermined. A topic shift in which it was evident that the speaker had switched topics but it was difficult to determine what the new topic was is called *undetermined.*

Topic shading and *topic initiation* were seen as continuous (Keenan & Schieffelin, 1976) or coherent (Crow, 1983), whereas the other types of topic shifts (e.g., *renewal, unexpected*) were seen as discontinuous (Keenan & Schieffelin, 1976) or noncoherent (Crow, 1983).

3. Reason for Shift

The classification of the reasons for shifting topics was far from exhaustive and the most difficult to determine. In this category, it was hoped that there would be superficial exploration of the intentions of the speakers as they shifted topics. Although the present research was not interested in directly examining nonverbal communication, these cues helped in interpreting a speaker's possible motivation for shifting topics. For example, a look of puzzlement may indicate a difficulty in comprehending what had just been said.

Some of these categories were almost all-inclusive. For instance, in *decreased comprehension* there was no distinction between problems with the delivery of the message and the identification of a referent—yet, these are totally different entities. It was felt that more detailed categorization would be even more difficult for analyzers to determine, whereas a general difficulty in comprehending was significantly different from other categories to be operational. Categories for classifying "Reason for Shift" follow here.

3.1. End of Topic. The topic shift had occurred because it was obvious that the speakers had nothing more to say about the previous topic. This might be signaled by a series of "passing" turns during which no more semantic information had been added, or following a period of silence.

3.2. Decreased Comprehension. It appeared from the observation of the videotape that the speaker had not fully comprehended what the other speaker had said and hence decided to change the topic. This might occur because the listener was not paying attention or because there was difficulty in identifying the referent or in understanding the gist of what was said (Keenan & Schieffelin, 1976). Decreased comprehension could also occur when there was difficulty in the delivery of the message.

3.3. Failure to Continue. A failure to continue occurred when a member of the dyad decided or could not continue a current unfinished topic forcing the other member of the dyad to change the topic.

3.4. Outside Event. A topic shift had occurred because of something that happened in the immediate environment (e.g., a telephone ringing) or an object/person in the immediate environment had triggered a new topic of conversation.

3.5. Repetition of an Idea. A topic shift had occurred because of a need to repeat a previously mentioned idea.

3.6. Anecdotal. A topic shift had occurred because of a desire to share a short story, usually biographical in nature.

3.7. Undetermined. The reason for the topic shift did not appear to fit into any of the categories mentioned previously.

4. Relation to Context

In categorizing the type of context to which a shift related, it was hoped that there would be some notion of the type of knowledge used in these conversations. For example, were subjects always shifting to information relating to the outside environment or did they relate more to specific knowledge that was shared? The categories used for context follow here:

4.1. Text. The topic shift related to something that was previously said in the conversation—knowledge that had already been shared.

4.2. Environment. The topic shift related to an object or event in the immediate environment (e.g., the tablecloth, someone who had just dropped something, etc.).

4.3. Specific Knowledge. The topic shift related to knowledge within the speaker(s)' repertoire (e.g., personal experiences).

4.4. General Knowledge. The topic shift related to knowledge assumed to be within the realm of the general public's repertoire (e.g., world events).

4.5. Unknown. The analyzers were unable to determine what the topic shift related to.

ACKNOWLEDGMENTS

This work was conducted by Linda J. Garcia in partial fulfillment of the requirements for the PhD in biomedical sciences (speech/language pathology) at Université de Montréal. The authors are grateful to Jean-Luc Nespoulous, Marcia Zuker, Caroline Bredeson, Jane McGarry, and Jennifer Platt for their help with this project.

REFERENCES

Austin, J. L. (1962). *How to do things with words.* Oxford: Clarendon.

Brinton, B., & Fujiki, M. (1984). Development of topic manipulation skills in discourse. *Journal of Speech and Hearing Research, 27,* 350–358.

Campbell-Taylor, I. (1984). *Dimensions of clinical judgment in the diagnosis of Alzheimer's disease.* Unpublished doctoral dissertation, State University of New York at Buffalo, NY.

Crow, B. (1983). Topic shifts in couples' conversations. In R. T. Craig & K. Tracy (Eds.), *Conversational coherence: Form, structure and strategy* (pp. 136–156). Beverly Hills, CA: Sage.

de Ajuriaguerra, J., & Tissot, R. (1975). Some aspects of language in various forms of senile dementia (comparisons with language in childhood). In E. H. Lenneberg & E. Lenneberg (Eds.), *Foundations of language development* (pp. 323–339). New York: Academic Press.

Dore, J. (1975). Holophrases, speech acts and language universals. *Journal of Child Language, 2,* 21–40.

Dore, J. (1979). Conversation and preschool language development. In P. Fletcher & M. Garman (Eds.), *Language acquisition* (pp. 337–361). New York: Cambridge University Press.

Ernst, B., Dalby, M. A., & Dalby, A. (1970). Aphasic disturbances in presenile dementia. *Acta Neurologica Scandinavica*, 41–47, 99–100.

Garcia, L., & Joanette, Y. (1994). *Conversational topic shifting profiles in dementia of the Alzheimer type: A multiple case study*. Manuscript submitted for review.

Goldberg, J. A. (1983). A move toward describing conversational coherence. In R. T. Craig & K. Tracy (Eds.), *Conversational coherence* (pp. 25–45). Beverly Hills, CA: Sage.

Goodenough, D. R., & Weiner, S. L. (1978). The role of conversational passing moves in the management of topical transitions. *Discourse Processes, 1*, 395–404.

Goodglass, H., & Kaplan, E. (1976). *The assessment of aphasia and related disorders*. Philadelphia: Lea & Febiger.

Grice, H. P. (1975). Logic and conversation. In P. Cole & J. L. Morgan (Eds.), *Syntax and semantics: Vol. 3: Speech acts* (pp. 41–58). New York: Academic Press.

Hegde, M. N. (1987). *Clinical research in communicative disorders: Principles and strategies*. Boston: College-Hill Press.

Holtgraves, T., Srull, T. K., & Socall, D. (1989). Conversation memory: The effects of speaker status on memory for the assertiveness of conversation remarks. *Journal of Personality and Social Psychology, 56*(2), 149–160.

Hutchinson, J. M., & Jensen, M. (1980). A pragmatic evaluation of discourse communication in normal and senile elderly in a nursing home. In L. K. Obler & M. L. Albert (Eds.), *Language and communication in the elderly* (pp. 59–73). Lexington, MA: D.C. Heath.

Illes, J. (1986). *The structure of spontaneous language production in Alzheimer's, Huntington's and Parkinson's Disease*. Unpublished doctoral dissertation, Stanford University, CA.

Illes, J. (1989). Neurolinguistic features of spontaneous language production dissociate three forms of neurodegenerative disease: Alzheimer's, Huntington's, and Parkinson's. *Brain and Language, 37*, 628–642.

Irigaray, L. (1967). Approche psycho-linguistique du langage des déments [A psycholinguistic approach to language in dementia]. *Neuropsychologia, 5*, 25–52.

Keenan, E. O., & Schieffelin, B. B. (1976). Topic as a discourse notion: A study of topic in the conversations of children and adults. In C. N. Li (Ed.), *Subject and topic* (pp. 337–384). New York: Academic Press.

Kintsch, W. (1988). The role of knowledge in discourse comprehension: A construction-integration model. *Psychological Review, 9*, 163–182.

Kintsch, W., & Van Dijk, T. A. (1978). Toward a model of text comprehension. *Psychological Review, 85*, 363–394.

Levinson, S. (1984). *Pragmatics*. Cambridge: Cambridge University Press.

Lorch, R. F., Lorch, E. P., & Matthews, P. D. (1985). On-line processing of the topic structure of a text. *Journal of Memory and Language, 24*, 350–362.

Lubinski, R. (1984). *Environmental considerations in working with the elderly*. Short course given in London, Ontario.

McKhann, G., Drachman, D., Folstein, M., Katzman, R., Price, D., & Stadlan, E. M. (1984). Clinical diagnosis of Alzheimer's disease. *Neurology, 34*, 939–944.

McLaughlin, M. L. (1984). *Conversation: How talk is organized*. Beverly Hills, CA: Sage.

McReynolds, L. V., & Kearns, K. P. (1983). *Single-subject experimental designs in communicative disorders*. Baltimore, MD: University Park Press.

Moeschler, J. (1993). Relevance and conversation. *Lingua, 90*, 149–171.

Murphy, G. L. (1990). The psycholinguistics of discourse comprehension. In Y. Joanette & H. H. Brownell (Eds.), *Discourse ability and brain damage: Theoretical and empirical perspectives* (pp. 28–49). New York: Springer-Verlag.

Obler, L. K. (1979). *Psycholinguistic aspects of language in dementia*. Paper presented in symposium on Language and Communication in Healthy and Dementing Elderly, Academy of Aphasia, San Diego, CA.

Obler, L. K., & Albert, M. L. (1981). Language and aging: A neurobehavioral analysis. In D. S. Beasley & G. A. Davis (Eds.), *Aging: Communication processes and disorders* (pp. 107–121). New York: Grune & Stratton.

Planalp, S., & Tracy, K. (1980). Not to change the topic but...: A cognitive approach to the management of conversation. In D. Nimmo (Ed.), *Communication yearbook 4* (pp. 237–258). New Brunswick, NJ: Transaction Books.

Reisberg, B., Ferris, S. H., De Leon, M. J., & Crook, T. (1982). The Global Deterioration Scale for assessment of primary degenerative dementia. *American Journal of Psychiatry, 139*, 9.

Revelation Technologies. (1987). *Advanced revelation*. Bellevue, WA: Author.

Ripich, D. N., & Terrell, B. Y. (1988). Patterns of discourse cohesion and coherence in Alzheimer's disease. *Journal of Speech and Hearing Disorders, 53*, 8–15.

Ripich, D. N., Terrell, B. Y., & Spinelli, F. (1983). Discourse cohesion in senile dementia of the Alzheimer type. In R. H. Brookshire (Ed.), *Clinical aphasiology conference proceedings* (pp. 316–321). Minneapolis: BRK Publishers.

Ripich, D. N., Vertes, D., Whitehouse, P., & Fulton, S. (1988). *Conversational discourse patterns in senile dementia of the Alzheimer's type patients*. Paper presented at the American Speech-Language-Hearing Association Annual Convention, Boston, MA.

Sanders, R. E. (1983). Tools for cohering discourse and their strategic utilization: Markers of structural connections and meaning relations. In R. T. Craig & K. Tracy (Eds.), *Conversational coherence: Form, structure, and strategy* (pp. 67–80). Beverly Hills, CA: Sage.

Searle, J. R. (1965). "What is a speech act?". In M. Black (Ed.), *Philosophy in America* (pp. 221–239). Cornell: Allen & Unwin.

Searle, J. R. (1969). *Speech acts: An essay in the philosophy of language*. New York: Cambridge University Press.

Searle, J. R. (1975). Indirect speech acts. In P. Cole & J. L. Morgan (Eds.), *Syntax and semantics: Vol. 3: Speech acts* (pp. 59–82). New York: Academic Press.

Tracy, K. (1982). On getting the point: Distinguishing "issues" from "events," an aspect of conversational coherence. In M. Burgoon (Ed.), *Communication yearbook 5* (pp. 279–301). New Brunswick, NJ: Transaction Books.

Tracy, K., & Moran, J. P., III. (1983). Conversational relevance in multiple-goal settings. In R. T. Craig & K. Tracy (Eds.), *Conversational coherence* (pp. 116–135). Beverly Hills, CA: Sage.

Van Dijk, T. A. (1977). Context and cognition: Knowledge frames and speech act comprehension. *Journal of Pragmatics, 1*, 211–232.

Van Dijk, T. A. (1980). *Macrostructures: An interdisciplinary study of global structures in discourse, interaction, and cognition*. Hillsdale, NJ: Lawrence Erlbaum Associates.

Van Dijk, T. A. (1981). *Studies in the pragmatics of discourse*. The Hague: Mouton Publishers.

Van Dijk, T. A., & Kintsch, W. (1983). *Strategies of discourse comprehension*. New York: Academic Press.

Wardhaugh, R. (1985). *How conversation works*. New York: Basil Blackwell.

Wilson, D., & Sperber, D. (1981). *On Grice's theory of conversation and discourse: Structure and interpretation*. New York: St. Martin's.

Chapter **11**

Requests for Clarification as Evidence of Pragmatic Comprehension Difficulty: The Case of Alzheimer's Disease

Heidi E. Hamilton
Georgetown University

One manifestation of Alzheimer's disease is a progressive and apparently irreversible deterioration of the patient's ability to communicate with others. Researchers generally agree that an Alzheimer's patient's problems in communication are due less to phonological and morphosyntactic disorders than to difficulties on the semantic and pragmatic levels (Appell, Kertesz, & Fisman, 1982; Bayles, 1979; Bayles & Kaszniak, 1987; Hier, Hagenlocker, & Shindler, 1985; Kempler, 1984; Obler, 1981; Schwartz, Marin, & Saffran, 1979). Because of their basically well-formed syntactic structure, most of the inappropriate or irrelevant utterances characteristic of the language used by Alzheimer's patients would not appear out of the ordinary in isolation (with the exception of neologisms), but only when heard within the larger discourse context in pursuit of some interactional goal. In line 3 of Example 1, the utterances "You can do that. That's a good idea," which are produced by an Alzheimer's patient, are perfectly well-formed syntactically but become marked in the larger discourse.

	1. Patient:	And where did you say your home was?	
	2. Researcher:	I'm on Walter Road.	
→	3. Patient:	You can do that. That's a good idea.	(1)

In such situations of communicative uncertainty, when a listener has difficulty in making sense of what the speaker has just said, he or she has several options. Goffman (1967) suggested that, when faced with such a situation, interlocutors use either an avoidance strategy or a corrective strategy. That is, a listener may immediately intervene with an other-initiated repair (see also Schegloff, Jefferson, & Sacks, 1977, on repair), often in the form of a request for clarification, to alleviate the confusion. Alternatively, a listener may just ride out the situation for a while, hoping that things will become clearer later in the interaction.

In addition to the two types of interactional strategies Goffman discussed, I have observed a type of hybrid strategy, as illustrated in Example 2. This strategy seems to straddle avoidance and correction. The speaker using this strategy makes a bow to the source of the sense-making trouble in what the previous speaker has just said by incorporating it into his or her next utterance, but immediately thereafter continues to say what he or she had initially wanted to say.

	1. Researcher:	Would you like a tissue for your nose? Would you like a Kleenex for your nose?
→	2. Patient:	(Mhm). Oh yes. *I know his name.*
→	3. Researcher:	*You know his name*, but can I get you a Kleenex for your nose? (2)

The researcher's repetition, *mutatis mutandis*, in line 3 of the patient's "I know his name" in line 2 neither *corrects* the barrier to sense-making in an explicit way (say, by asking "Whose name?" or "What do you mean?") nor *avoids* the barrier by simply repeating the initial question in lines 1 and 2 ("Would you like a tissue for your nose? Would you like a Kleenex for your nose?"), but makes an effortless link to the patient's utterance before allowing the researcher to get on with his or her own interactional goals (getting the patient to accept a tissue).[1]

Because of the variety of options open to interlocutors faced with barriers to understanding in conversation (and because neither analysts nor participants in conversations can read minds), we cannot know every interactional moment that may cause problems in sense-making for a listener. We can, however, investigate those cases in which a listener uses a corrective strategy in the form of a request for clarification. It is to this examination of these trouble sources as identified by interactional participants themselves that we now turn.

This chapter examines sense-making difficulties in 13 naturally occurring conversations I held with one elderly female Alzheimer's patient over the

---

[1]Note the phonological similarity between "nose" and "know his."

Which of these strategies is chosen to respond to sense-making difficulties seems to be influenced by the primary function of a given chunk of talk as perceived by the speaker. If the speaker perceives understanding to be more important than face issues in the interaction, he or she can take actions to correct the misunderstanding by issuing an other-initiated repair (Schegloff et al., 1977). If the speaker perceives face issues to be more important than the understanding of a proposition in the situation, she or he can avoid talking about the misunderstanding. The response strategies then can be understood as being motivated by the intricate intertwining of the goals of coherence, positive face maintenance (relating to the individual's need to be liked and to have his or her wishes understood), and negative face maintenance (relating to an individual's need for independence; see Brown & Levinson, 1987, for a discussion of positive and negative face; for a more detailed discussion of response strategies see Hamilton, 1991).

4½-year period between November 1981 and March 1986 in a private health-care center. As just discussed, it is often difficult to determine whether these sense-making problems belong solely to the analyst (although I was also a participant) looking in from the outside at the interactions or whether they were experienced by the interlocutors themselves at the time of the interactions. As one way of dealing with this uncertainty, I decided to focus on those areas of the discourse that are attempts by the participants themselves to clear away trouble sources to sense-making in the conversations. An examination of the participants' requests for clarification of each other's utterances can provide us with important information "straight from the horse's mouth" regarding problems in the sense-making process as the participants identify them.

At the time of the interactions examined here, the patient, who will be called Elsie Smith, was 81–86 years old.[2] Elsie Smith had earned an advanced degree and had been professionally active as a leader in the church until retiring 10 years prior to the beginning of this study. She had an outgoing personality and was very friendly to residents, volunteers, and staff alike. Elsie enjoyed taking part in social activities and was visibly pleased when she saw people she recognized at these activities. According to the Global Deterioration Scale (GDS) for age-associated cognitive decline and Alzheimer's disease (Reisberg, Ferris, de Leon et al., 1982), she was at Stage 5, moderately severe cognitive decline, at the onset of our conversations in 1981 and had reached Stage 7, very severe cognitive decline, by 1986. At the beginning of the study, Elsie Smith could walk and eat independent of others' assistance; by 1985 she needed assistance to eat and drink. By March 1986, she was bedridden and her verbal production consisted of the responses "mmm," "mhm," "mm hm," "hmm?", and "uhhuh," although her systematic use of these indicates some comprehension on her part, especially of personally important topics (see Hamilton, 1994). The appendix provides prose characterizations of Elsie's general communicative abilities at various points along the progression of the disease.

TYPES OF CLARIFICATION REQUESTS

Using the categories of clarification requests discussed in McTear (1985) based on Garvey (1977, 1979), 279 requests for clarification were identified in the 13 conversations: 155 issued by me; 124 by Elsie. Examples 3–8 illustrate these 6 categories of clarification requests as they occurred in the data. Table 11.1 provides a summary of the use of the various types of clarification requests by

[2]I wish to thank Ms. Jill Bergen, Coordinator of Volunteer Services, The Hermitage in Northern Virginia, for arranging permission for me to tape record interactions in which I was involved as a volunteer, and Elsie Smith, a remarkable woman whom I never saw only as an informant but came to love as a friend.

TABLE 11.1
Elsie's Clarification Requests (n = 124)

	NR	*SR*	*SC*	*SS*	*PE*	*PC*	*Totals*
1981	4 (8%)	0	13 (28%)	5 (11%)	14 (30%)	11 (23%)	47
1982	14 (23%)	3 (5%)	22 (35%)	3 (5%)	2 (3%)	18 (29%)	62
1984	5 (83%)	0	0	0	0	1 (17%)	6
1985	4 (67%)	0	1 (17%)	0	0	1 (17%)	6
1986	3 (100%)	0	0	0	0	0	3
	30 (24%)	3 (2%)	36 (29%)	8 (6%)	16 (13%)	31 (25%)	124

Note. NR = nonspecific request for repetition (e.g., "What?," "Huh?")
SR = specific request for repetition (e.g. "Quite a few of what?")
SC = specific request for confirmation (e.g., "In that green one?")
SS = specific request for specification (e.g., "Who [will be all right]?")
PE = potential request for elaboration (e.g., "And what . . . which time?")
PC = potential request for confirmation (e.g., "Today you mean?")

Elsie over the 4 ½-year time period; Table 11.2 provides the same summary of my use of clarification requests over the same time period.

Example 3 illustrates a nonspecific request for repetition (NR). The requester's goal is to cause the conversational partner to repeat the entire utterance that prompted the request for clarification.[3]

1. Heidi: Is he new here?
→ 2. Elsie: What?
3. Heidi: Is he new here? Has he just started working
4. here?
5. Elsie: Oh maybe. I yeah..I don't know. . . (3)

In line 2, Elsie asks "What?" to which I respond in line 3 with a repetition of line 1 followed by a paraphrase of that utterance.

Example 4 illustrates a specific request for repetition (SR). The requester's goal in this case is to cause the conversational partner to repeat a specific word or words from the utterance that prompted the request for clarification.

1. Elsie: Did they have quite a few of the (lattice)?
→ 2. Heidi: Quite a few of what?
3. Elsie: Yeah. Oh good. Good. (4)

[3] Transcription conventions by Tannen (1984):
[Brackets between lines indicate overlapping speech
[Two people talking at the same time
Brackets on two lines]
] indicate second utterance latched onto first without a perceptible pause

TABLE 11.2
Heidi's Clarification Requests (n = 155)

	NR	*SR*	*SC*	*SS*	*PE*	*PC*	*Totals*
1981	0	1 (100%)	0	0	0	0	1
1982	0	1 (4%)	17 (65%)	6 (23%)	0	2 (8%)	26
1984	6 (14%)	9 (21%)	17 (40%)	8 (19%)	2 (4%)	1 (2%)	43
1985	24 (32%)	13 (17%)	25 (33%)	4 (5%)	7 (9%)	3 (4%)	76
1986	4 (44%)	0	5 (56%)	0	0	0	9
	34 (22%)	24 (15%)	64 (41%)	18 (12%)	9 (6%)	6 (4%)	155

Note. NR = nonspecific request for repetition (e.g., "What?," "Huh?")
SR = specific request for repetition (e.g. "Quite a few of what?")
SC = specific request for confirmation (e.g., "In that green one?")
SS = specific request for specification (e.g., "Who [will be alright]?")
PE = potential request for elaboration (e.g., "And what . . . which time?")
PC = potential request for confirmation (e.g., "Today you mean?")

In line 2, I ask "Quite a few of what?" expecting to get a repetition of the portion of line 1 that I did not hear. In this case, Elsie did not respond to the request as I had expected, giving me instead an affirmative response to a wh-question (see Hamilton, 1994, for a discussion of the qualitative changes in Elsie's types of inappropriate responses to questions).

Example 5 illustrates a specific request for confirmation (SC). The requester's goal in this case is to cause the conversational partner to respond affirmatively or negatively to the requester's rephrasing or repetition of the utterance that prompted the request for clarification.

	1. Elsie:	So it they have some special things in that	
	2.	little cab there. I don't know (it is)	
→	3. Heidi:	[in that green one?	
	4. Elsie:	Yes, this white yes little whitish one there. . .	(5)

In line 3, I rephrase Elsie's utterance "in that little cab there" as "in that green one?" and ask for her agreement that I have understood what she meant in lines 1 and 2. In this case, Elsie appears in line 4 to agree with my paraphrase ("yes") but makes a change in identifying color from green to white.

Example 6 illustrates a specific request for specification (SS). The requester's goal is for the conversational partner to provide further specification of some item mentioned in the utterance that prompted the request for clarification.

	1. Elsie:	But here I think he'll be alright.	
→	2. Heidi:	Who?	
	3. Elsie:	That was one of the (frien) one (wemb) member.	(6)

In line 2, I use "who?" to ask for further specification of the pronoun "he" as used by Elsie in line 1. In line 3, she complies (albeit somewhat vaguely) with my request for clarification by providing some additional identifying information.

The potential requests illustrated in Examples 7 and 8 differ from their specific counterparts illustrated in Examples 5 and 6 in that the potential requests focus on an element that is missing from the surface form of the prompt but that is "potentially available" according to Garvey (1977). The specific requests, on the other hand, focus on an element that is already part of the surface form of the prompt, but that is for some reason not specific enough for the listener's needs.

Example 7 illustrates a potential request for elaboration (PE). The requester's goal here is to cause the conversational partner to provide information not included in the utterance that prompted the request for clarification.

	1. Heidi:	We're going to exercise class.	
→	2. Elsie:	And what. .which time?	
	3. Heidi:	Right now.	(7)

In line 2, Elsie asks me to indicate *when* "we're going to exercise class," which I then do in line 3.

Example 8 illustrates a potential request for confirmation (PC). The requester's goal here is to cause the conversational partner to respond affirmatively or negatively to the requester's guessed-at extension of the verb complement in the utterance that prompted the request for clarification.

	1. Heidi:	Do you have your red book somewhere?	
→	2. Elsie:	Today [you mean?	
	3. Heidi:	[yeah is it?	
	4. Elsie:	Oh let me see whether I have it.	(8)

In line 2, Elsie guesses that I mean "today" in my utterance in line 1, although I do not say so explicitly. After hearing that I agree with her guess (line 3), Elsie responds in line 4 to my question represented in line 1.

DISCUSSION OF THE FINDINGS

An examination of Elsie's and my use of clarification requests in conversations with each other over 4½ years as represented in Tables 11.1 and 11.2 reveals that (a) Elsie produces markedly fewer requests for clarification over time as the Alzheimer's disease progresses, and (b) Elsie's and my relative use of potential requests for confirmation (PC) differs significantly.

With regard to the first point, we note in Table 11.1 the overall decline in Elsie's use of clarification requests (except for nonspecific requests for repetition like "huh" and "what?") in 1984 and beyond. Of Elsie's 124 requests for clarification, 109 take place before 1984. Of the 15 requests for clarification in the period 1984–1986, only 3 are not of the nonspecific type. This decline in substantive requests for clarification suggests that Elsie seems essentially to have lost the ability at that point to assess her own comprehension ability and needs. This interpretation is corroborated by other communicative behaviors on Elsie's part during these interactions. For example, at the time of Elsie's marked decrease in requests for clarification, we note that Elsie stops providing accounts (Scott & Lyman, 1968) in the form of excuses and justifications for her forgetfulness and inability to carry out basic tasks, such as remembering her children's names. The use of such excuses and justifications may indicate that the account-giver realizes his or her behavior does not match the conversational partner's expectations of him or her. Elsie's lack of accounts at the later stages of the disease provides additional evidence that she has a decreasing understanding of what her conversational partner expects of her. Additionally, at this approximate stage in her disease, Elsie also stops referring to her memory problems (e.g., "I forget.") and stops providing explicit linguistic evaluations of her own performance at a given time (e.g., "We're coming along alright"; "I can do an awful lot").

With regard to the second point just mentioned, by comparing Tables 11.1 and 11.2, we note Elsie's significantly greater use of the potential request for confirmation as compared with my use of this type. Whereas 31 of 124 (25%) of Elsie's total number of requests for clarification are potential requests for confirmation, only 6 of 155 (4%) of my total number of requests for clarification are of this type.[4] When we look at representative illustrations of Elsie's use of requests for potential confirmation (Examples 8, 9, and 10), there appears to be a clash of expectations between Elsie's comprehension of my utterances (which prompts her requests for clarification) and my own design of those utterances. Consider Example 8 again: A temporal adverb ("now" or "today") was not initially provided in the question in line 1; Elsie apparently needed it, as evidenced by her request for clarification in line 2.

	1. Heidi:	Do you have your red book somewhere?	
→	2. Elsie:	Today [you mean?	
	3. Heidi:	[yeah is it?	
	4. Elsie:	Oh let me see whether I have it.	(8)

[4]Even if we limit our investigation to the use of requests for clarification in 1981–1982 (due to the marked decline in overall use of such requests by Elsie between 1984–1986 as evidenced in Table 11.1), we find that potential requests for confirmation (PC) comprise 29 of 109 (27%) of Elsie's requests for clarification as contrasted with 2 of 27 (4%) of my requests for clarification.

Likewise, in Example 9, temporal and spatial adverbs ("now" and "here") were not initially provided in the statement in line 1; again Elsie apparently needed these references, as evidenced by her requests for clarification in lines 2, 5, and 7.

	1. Heidi:	I just came to talk. [
→	2. Elsie:	[oh good. [You gonna be here
	3. Heidi:	[What do you have
	4.	there?
→	5. Elsie:	You gonna be here (for right) now?
	6. Heidi:	Uhhuh.
→	7. Elsie:	Right here?
	8. Heidi:	Uhhuh.
	9. Elsie:	This way?
	10. Heidi:	Yeah. I just came to talk to you. That's all. [
	11. Elsie:	[Oh
	12.	that's good. Thank you, dear honey. (9)

Similarly, in Example 10, the spatial adverb "here" was not provided when reference was made in line 1 to the necklace Elsie was wearing at the time.

	1. Heidi:	This is a nice necklace that you have.
→	2. Elsie:	Here?
	3. Heidi:	The. .the necklace here.
	4. Elsie:	Oh yes. (10)

Elsie's request for clarification in line 2 indicates that she was missing that information in my utterance represented in line 1.

What is the possible significance of Elsie's greater use of potential requests for confirmation when compared with mine? I would like to suggest that Sperber and Wilson's (1986; Wilson & Sperber, 1984) work on relevance can shed some light on this problem. In their discussion of Grice (1975) in which Grice argued that listeners are able to infer speaker meaning based on speaker deviations from maxims of quality ("be truthful"), quantity ("be sufficiently informative"), relevance ("be relevant"), and manner ("be concise"), Wilson and Sperber (1984) noted that "merely instructing speakers to make their utterances relevant would constrain them hardly at all" and consequently added the notion of degrees of relevance. It is therefore not enough for speakers just to be relevant; they need to be as relevant as possible. According to Sperber and Wilson, listeners operate according to the principle of relevance in the interpretation of every utterance (i.e., listeners assume "that the speaker has tried to be as relevant as possible in the circumstances"). In comparing the relevance of propositions, Sperber and Wilson utilized the notion of efficiency or processing effort, which, in turn, is determined by three main factors: (a) complexity of the utterance, (b) size of the context, and (c) accessibility of the context. The greater the processing effort a proposition requires, the less relevant it will be in a given situation. A speaker aiming at maximal relevance should, among other things, make sure that his or her utterance is more easily accessible to the listener than any other utterance he or she could have produced in the circumstances.

According to Sperber and Wilson's insights, then, I had designed my utterances to Elsie as represented in line 1 of Examples 8, 9, and 10 with the idea that her effort to process these utterances would be minimal (i.e., that the utterances I produced would be more easily accessible to her than any other utterances I could have produced in those circumstances). I assumed explicit reference to the "here and now" to be unnecessary unless something in the context had made a reference to another time and place more easily accessible to Elsie. It appears from Examples 8–10 and many others like them in the database, however, that Elsie needed greater specification of the verb complement than that with which I provided her in the prompts.

Wilson and Sperber (1984) suggested that such mismatches in expectations between speaker and listener are due to the fact that "the speaker has failed to notice, and hence eliminate, an interpretation that was both accessible enough to the hearer and productive enough in terms of contextual implications to be accepted without question" (p. 33). The situation represented in Examples 8–10 does seem to be different, however, from the situations one normally thinks of when dealing with accessibility of a particular speaker, meaning those based, for example, on lexical ambiguity, as illustrated by the constructed Example 11. The lexical item "hot" could in certain contexts be interpreted as referring either to the temperature of the food or its degree of spiciness.

This food isn't hot enough. (11)

Whereas it could be argued that greater specificity would be necessary in certain contexts to disambiguate the lexical item "hot," thereby eliminating the listener's confusion as to the most relevant, accessible speaker meaning in Example 11, a more complete specification of the verb complement in the cases shown in Examples 8–10 would seem to be uneconomical and inefficient, and in most cases unnecessary.

Wilson and Sperber (1984) maintained that the principle of relevance does not vary from situation to situation and culture to culture, but instead has its origins in very general constraints on human cognition. How do we then account for the apparent mismatch of expectations regarding what counts as relevant as evidenced in Examples 8–10? Wilson and Sperber suggested that what does vary is the stock of assumptions that listeners can draw on in the interpretation process, the accessibility of these assumptions, and the amount of processing effort they are prepared to expend. They go on to suggest that "pragmatic variation might provide some interesting indirect evidence on the organization of memory, the accessibility of assumptions and the allocation of processing resources" (pp. 40–41).

In this sense, Elsie's significantly greater proportion of potential requests for confirmation of information that arguably was unnecessary to a normal understanding of speaker meaning (indicating her difficulty in processing what would seem to be an easily accessible meaning), suggests that she may have some difficulty with pragmatic comprehension (comprehension of speaker meaning as opposed to the comprehension of the semantic meaning of individual lexical items or sentences).

This finding is interesting to consider because one of Elsie's major communicative difficulties had earlier (Hamilton, 1991) been identified as being her lack of ability to interpret indirect discourse in its indirect meaning (i.e., to figure out what a speaker means—pragmatic meaning—when that underlying meaning differs from what the speaker is actually saying on the propositional or semantic level). Example 12 illustrates Elsie's difficulty in interpreting my (extreme) use of indirectness that is fueled in this situation in part by my reluctance to say explicitly to Elsie that I felt I needed to leave her and visit other residents. Just prior to the segment in Example 12, I had helped Elsie back to her room from the lounge where we had been talking for approximately 30 minutes.

1. Elsie: Please sit down.
2. Heidi: Oh well, that's okay. I think I should probably
3. go and see some more people, but I wanted to come
4. and talk with you this morning.
5. Elsie: Oh you mean, wait a minute. What what did you
6. say?
7. Heidi: I I just said that I should probably go and see
8. a couple more people before exercise class starts.
9. Elsie: Oh. for today
10. Heidi: uhhuh. for today. and then I'll
11. be back for you when the class starts if you want
12. to join us for exercise.
13. Elsie: oh you mean oh you oh I see
14. Heidi: Uhhuh.
15. Elsie: You mean then to look for us. Is that what you
16. meant?
17. Heidi: I came to talk to you this morning
18. Elsie: mhm
19. Heidi: because I think you're so interesting.
20. Elsie: Well, you're glad that you can stay as long as

21. you want to stay a while.
22. Heidi: Okay.
23. Elsie: Yes. (—?—)
24. Heidi: You've got
25. Elsie: You can sit right here.
26. Heidi: such interesting things. Okay.
27. Elsie: You sit right there. (12)

Example 12 exhibits Elsie's difficulties in deciphering my very indirect refusal (lines 2–4, 7–8) of her invitation for me to sit down (line 1) in her room. My reluctance to say "no" directly to her prompted her to ask me several times what I meant (lines 5–6, 13, 15–16), resulting, humorously enough, in a change in my plans. I ended up accepting Elsie's reissued invitation (lines 20–21, 25, 27) to stay and talk with her, and I visited the other residents later in the day.

Of course, the difficulty on the part of the patient in understanding speaker meaning in cases of indirect discourse as illustrated by Example 12 is a more obvious and expected phenomenon (because of the greater processing effort required by the listener to interpret indirect discourse) than that which I argue is evidenced by her high proportion of use of potential requests for confirmation as indicated in Examples 8–10.

SUMMARY

An examination of 279 requests for clarification in 13 naturally occurring conversations I had with one Alzheimer's patient over 4½ years—with regard to overall use over time as well as with regard to the relative use of 6 different types of such requests—led me to make two points. First, that decreased use of requests for clarification over time by the patient provides us with explicit linguistic evidence of the patient's decreasing ability to assess her own comprehension ability and needs. This observation was supported by the patient's decreasing production of accounts, decreasing references to memory problems, and decreasing self-evaluations. Second, that the patient's significantly greater use of potential requests for confirmation (as compared with my use of the same type of request) of information that arguably is unnecessary to a normal understanding of speaker meaning (such as explicit reference to the "here and now") provides evidence of difficulty with pragmatic comprehension that may be a precursor to other documented forms of pragmatic difficulty, such as problems in understanding indirect discourse.

It is hoped that future research based on the observations made here about the patient's decreasing ability over time to assess her own comprehension ability and needs and her difficulty in understanding different types of speaker meaning will prove to be useful both to theoretical issues of linguistic pragmatics and to issues of importance to clinicians and other persons caring for Alzheimer's patients. Such insights may (a) provide us with information as to the possible linguistic manifestations of pragmatic breakdown over time and the hierarchical ordering of these manifestations; (b) suggest parameters of tasks based on the degree and sequencing of pragmatic decline that might be successfully used in clinical assessments of the progression of Alzheimer's disease; and (c) provide healthy interlocutors with clues as how best to accommodate the difficulties Alzheimer's patients may bring with them to interactions. It could be, for example, that a healthy speaker's explicit reference to the "here and now" (in those cases where this reference would normally be understood without being stated) will help an Alzheimer's patient understand more quickly what is meant, thereby preempting the need for requests for clarification of this type of information. Certainly the findings of this study suggest that attempts by healthy interlocutors to reduce the amount of inferencing an Alzheimer's patient must do (by being both explicit and direct) could result in increased understanding of propositional content on the part of the patient. As with most things, however, this benefit has its costs. The very directness that may serve to increase a patient's understanding may cause that same patient to feel talked down to, bossed around, or yelled at (see Tannen, 1984, for a discussion of the face-saving aspects of indirectness in conversation). Studies focusing on the effectiveness of a variety of discourse strategies in promoting both increased understanding and increased general well-being in conversations with Alzheimer's patients are a necessary next step in the interactional sociolinguistic approach taken in this study to the complex relationships between language use and Alzheimer's disease.

APPENDIX: PROSE CHARACTERIZATION OF FOUR STAGES OF ELSIE'S COMMUNICATIVE ABILITIES

Stage 1: Active, Confused, and Aware (ca. 1981–1982)

In this first stage of our interactions, Elsie is a very active participant both in terms of proportion of total number of words produced and in terms of proportion of total number of questions asked in each conversation. She is having trouble finding words in conversation, but more frequently deals with this problem by providing a circumlocution or a semantically related word rather than a neologism, a word with a completely different lexical meaning, or an empty word, as she does later. Elsie is also having to deal with her problem in tracking and producing referents for full noun phrases, although this is not evidenced in the very beginning of this stage. She is generally aware of her memory problems at this time, as evidenced by her explicit reference to them. She seems to be aware of the unusualness of these problems with word-finding, reference, and memory, as she often provides excuses (although they are generally insufficient) for this unexpected behavior. She also recognizes when her abilities are unexpectedly good as she provides explicit attests to these abilities and seems to be proud of them.

Elsie makes use of yes–no questions, including tag questions, as well as of a full range of wh-questions to ask about the past, present, and future. She refers with her questions to persons, objects, and events both within and beyond her sight. Her inappropriate responses to questions are primarily grammatically mismatched and vague responses as compared with structural-level inappropriate responses or nonresponses. She uses a good deal of idiosyncractic ready-made language in the design of her conversational contributions, including the marked use of opposites, the marked use of the conditional mood (although not until later phases of this stage), and her own professional language from earlier in her life. Despite some of the difficulties just mentioned, people generally enjoy talking with Elsie during this time. Contributing to this overall ease in talk seem to be Elsie's use of positive politeness devices, such as compliments, expressions of appreciation to others, terms of endearment, and lighthearted jokes.

Stage 2: Active, Confused, and Unaware (ca. 1984)

In Stage 2, Elsie continues to be an active participant in terms of proportion of total number of words produced in the conversations, but is much less active in producing questions in the interactions as compared with the first stage. It is more difficult to talk with Elsie now. This difficulty seems to stem in part from her decreasing awareness of her own communicative needs and those of others. In response to her word-finding problems, she no longer provides circumlocutions or semantically related words, but instead provides a neologism, an empty word, or a semantically unrelated word, options that are more difficult to "decode." Elsie no longer refers to her memory problems, nor does she provide excuses for her unexpected behavior. Her reference problems continue. She is beginning to repeat herself excessively (perseveration); when she does, the repetition generally is of whole clauses.

In terms of question production, Elsie continues to produce yes–no questions, including tag questions, and wh-questions (although no questions ask "who," "when," or "why"). The temporal reference of these questions continues to be to the past, present, and the future, although the spatial reference is now only to persons, objects, and events within sight. Her inappropriate responses tend to be relatively evenly distributed among response types, although the proportion of responses deemed inappropriate because of being vague or grammatically mismatched is somewhat lower, and the proportion of structural-level inappropriateness is higher, than in Stage 1. Elsie continues to use devices of positive politeness to make her conversational partner feel good, such as giving compliments, expressing appreciation, and telling jokes. She continues to make great use of the ready-made language she used in Stage 1.

Stage 3: Less Active, Confused, Unaware (ca. 1985)

In Stage 3, Elsie's participation in the conversations is markedly reduced, in terms of proportion both of total number of words and of question production, when compared with the first two stages. She continues to respond to her word-finding difficulties by using neologisms, empty words, and semantically unrelated words. She continues to have difficulty with reference. In terms of question production, Elsie no longer produces tag questions; the yes–no questions and wh-questions she uses (only "what?", "how?", and "which?") refer only to the present time. The inappropriateness of her responses now is largely due to "nonresponse." She frequently repeats herself and others excessively (perseveration), often involving the repetition of a single lexical item, although at times she still uses self- and other-repetition appropriately. She continues to use questions appropriately to ask for clarification and occasionally repairs her own utterances. Ready-made language continues to be used in the design of her conversational contributions. Most of the evidence of positive politeness (with the exception of the terms of endearment) that made talking with Elsie pleasant despite sense-making difficulties in the earlier stages are nowhere to be found in her discourse at this stage. Elsie no longer compliments or expresses interest in her conversational partner, nor does she express appreciation explicitly, use humor, or exclamatory questions. Elsie continues to be able to use attention-getting techniques, request action from her conversational partner, state her own wishes, check her own understanding, make statements about some of her disabilities, express deference, and use metacommunicative framing utterances.

Stage 4: Passive (ca. 1986)

In this stage, Elsie's participation level is even more markedly reduced than in Stage 3. Now she produces no lexical items, her utterances being confined to the set of "uhhuh," "mhm," "mm hm," "mmm," and "hmm?". Elsie's responses to questions, then, are either appropriate if an affirmative answer or an action would be considered appropriate, or inappropriate because of nonresponse or question-type mismatch (affirmative answer to a wh-question). Despite her limited communicative repertoire, Elsie is still able to request repetition of her conversational partner's utterance ("hmm?"), to take conversational turns appropriately, and to indicate that she recognizes personally important topics ("mmm" and by specific actions).

REFERENCES

Appell, J., Kertesz, A., & Fisman, M. (1982). A study of language functioning in Alzheimer patients. *Brain and Language, 17*, 73–91.

Bayles, K. A. (1979). *Communication profiles in a geriatric population.* Unpublished doctoral dissertation, University of Arizona, Tucson.

Bayles, K. A., & Kaszniak, A. (1987). *Communication and cognition in normal aging and dementia*. Boston: Little, Brown.

Brown, P., & Levinson, S. (1987). *Politeness: Some universals in language usage*. Cambridge: Cambridge University Press.

Garvey, C. (1977). The contingent query: A dependent act in conversation. In M. Lewis & L. Rosenblum (Eds.), *The origins of behavior* (pp. 63–94). New York: Wiley.

Garvey, C. (1979). Contingent queries and their relations in discourse. In E. Ochs & B. Schieffelin (Eds.), *Developmental pragmatics* (pp. 363–372). New York: Academic Press.

Goffman, E. (1967). On face-work. In E. Goffman (Ed.), *Interaction ritual* (pp. 5–45). Garden City: Doubleday.

Grice, P. (1975). Logic and conversation. In P. Cole & J. L. Morgan (Eds.), *Speech acts, syntax and semantics* (Vol. 3, pp. 41–58). New York: Academic Press.

Hamilton, H. (1991). Accommodation and mental disability. In H. Giles, N. Coupland, & J. Coupland (Eds.), *Contexts of accommodation: Developments in applied sociolinguistics* (pp. 157–186). Cambridge: Cambridge University Press.

Hamilton, H. (1994). *Conversations with an Alzheimer's patient*. Cambridge: Cambridge University Press.

Hier, D. B., Hagenlocker, K., & Shindler, A. G. (1985). Language disintegration in dementia: Effects of etiology and severity. *Brain and Language, 25*, 117–133.

Kempler, D. (1984). *Syntactic and symbolic abilities in Alzheimer's disease*. Unpublished doctoral dissertation, University of California, Los Angeles.

McTear, M. (1985). *Children's conversation*. Oxford: Basil Blackwell.

Obler, L. (1981). Review of *Le langage des dements* by Luce Irigaray. *Brain and Language, 12*, 375–386.

Reisberg, B., Ferris, S. H., de Leon, M. J., & Crook, J. (1982). The global deterioration scale (GDS): An instrument for the assessment of primary degenerative dementia (PDD). *American Journal of Psychiatry, 139*, 1136–1139.

Schegloff, E., Jefferson, G., & Sacks, H. (1977). The preference for self-correction in the organization of repair in conversation. *Language, 53*, 361–382.

Schwartz, M. F., Marin, O. S. M., & Saffran, E. M. (1979). Dissociations of language function in dementia: A case study. *Brain and Language, 7*, 277–306.

Scott, M., & Lyman, S. (1968). Accounts. *American Sociological Review, 33*(1), 46–62.

Sperber, D., & Wilson, D. (1986). *Relevance*. Cambridge, MA: Harvard University Press.

Tannen, D. (1984). *Conversational style*. Norwood, NJ: Ablex.

Wilson, D., & Sperber, D. (1984). Pragmatics: An overview. In S. George (Ed.), *From the linguistic to the social context* (pp. 21–41). Bologna: CLUEB.

Chapter 12

Cohesive Devices and Conversational Discourse in Alzheimer's Disease

Susan De Santi
New York University Medical Center

Laura Koenig
Loraine K. Obler
The City University of New York Graduate School

Joan Goldberger
The Parker Jewish Geriatric Center

Study of discourse of individuals with Alzheimer's disease has revealed much about the communicative abilities of those with this disease. In the early stages, a patient's discourse is characterized by vague responses and lexical imprecision. As a result, the listener does not quite know what the Alzheimer's patient is trying to say. With progression of the disease, discourse becomes increasingly disjointed until it is so disorganized that meaningful sequences cannot be produced (Bayles, Tomoeda, & Caffrey, 1982; Hamilton, chapter 11, this volume; Obler & Albert, 1984).

A variety of discourse abilities, including object description, picture description, picture narratives, interviews, and open-ended conversations have been examined, revealing a complex picture of discourse behavior in Alzheimer's disease. The descriptive discourse (e.g., describing an object) of mild-to-moderate Alzheimer's disease tends to be perseverative (Bayles, Tomoeda, Kaszniak, Stern, & Eagans, 1985), and this tendency increases with disease progression. Production of vague words and an increased reliance on indefinite terms were also noted on object description (Bayles, 1985). In picture descriptions, an increased number of empty phrases (phrases with little or no content; Nicholas, Obler, Albert, & Helm-Estabrooks, 1985), inappropriate use of anaphora (Hier, Hagenlocker, & Shindler, 1985), and reduction in the total number of words as well as the total number of unique words (Hier et al., 1985) have been observed. In addition, excessive verbosity with reduced information was displayed as the disease advanced.

Narrative discourse has also been examined in mild-to-moderate Alzheimer's disease using a picture story task (Ehrlich, 1990). In this study, each subject was given four different stories to narrate. The format of the pictorial display (narrative depicted in one picture frame and three picture frames) and the amount of content (two levels of story content designed where the second level included more information than the first) were manipulated. In general, the Alzheimer's subjects produced fewer propositions and total number of lexical items and more errors in anaphora than the normal control subjects. Further, more sentence fragments and shorter sentences distinguished the stories of the Alzheimer's group from those of the normal controls.

Numerous aspects of conversational discourse have been studied in Alzheimer's disease. For example, Hamilton (in press; chapter 11, this volume) longitudinally examined the ability of one Alzheimer's patient to request clarification of information during conversation with a researcher. As the disease progressed, the patient requested information less frequently from the conversation partner.

Ripich, Vertes, Whitehouse, Fulton, and Ekelman (1991) explored conversational turn-taking abilities, speech acts, and word usage during a dialogue between an Alzheimer's patient and an examiner. Patients with Alzheimer's disease, more often than normal control subjects, used fewer words per conversational turn, more nonverbal responses, and a greater number of unintelligible utterances. The most common type of speech act for the Alzheimer's group was requestives (e.g., "Do you drink tea?"), whereas the control group used more assertives (e.g., "I'll get some now"). Topic shifting in the conversation of 10 subjects (5 patients with Alzheimer's disease and 5 normal controls) with an examiner is reported on by Garcia and Joanette (chapter 10, this volume). The authors observed that the Alzheimer's patients seemed to change topic abruptly and had difficulty relating the new topic to the old. As a result, their discourse appeared to lack coherence.

In an assessment of topic-related interviews, Ripich and Terrell (1988) examined propositions, cohesive devices, and coherence of discourse in Alzheimer's disease. Of interest to us is the particular cohesive devices used by the Alzheimer's patients. In their study, no statistically significant difference between the percent of cohesive devices (categorized as *semantic* and *structural*) used by the Alzheimer's group and the normal control group was found. This held true for both appropriate and inappropriate use of cohesion. Ripich and Terrell reported their nonsignificant findings as trends. Structural cohesion, they said, was "slightly more frequent in the discourse of the AD [Alzheimer's] group" (24.4%) than in the normal control group (23.9%), whereas "semantic cohesion occurred somewhat less frequently in the AD group" (51.4% Alzheimer's group vs. 65.8% control group). In any event, although use of cohesive devices was statistically unremarkable in the Alzheimer's group, their discourse was judged by trained listeners to be markedly less coherent (determined by listener confusion) than that of the control group. This finding is important because it indicates that appropriate production of cohesive devices does not necessarily result in coherent discourse.

It is surprising that Ripich and Terrell found no statistical differences in the occurrence of cohesion between the groups studied. The distinction between structural and semantic cohesion is a useful one that should account for the differences observed between the form and the content of sentences spoken by the Alzheimer's group. Basically, we anticipated that sentence structure and the use of structural cohesion would be unremarkable in Alzheimer's disease, whereas semantic problems, which are abundant in this population, should manifest themselves through errors in semantic cohesion. We suspected that more refined definitions of structural and semantic cohesion would better capture the range of cohesive devices available to a speaker and might reveal group differences. For example, the Ripich and Terrell classification of semantic cohesion included categories such as reference, conjunction, and ellipsis. Another type of semantic cohesion, such as lexical cohesion (reproducing a previous item said by oneself or the interlocutor by using the same word, a homonym, a superordinate, etc.), could have been included in the analysis. We observed that by omitting analysis of lexical cohesion, a potentially important indicator of cohesive breakdown in Alzheimer's disease had been ignored, because lexical abilities are known to be compromised in the discourse of Alzheimer's disease (see Bayles & Kaszniak, 1987, for a review). Additionally, Ripich and Terrell (1988) included as structural cohesive devices units that maintained conversation but added no meaning to the discourse (e.g., "Well, uh, now, uh," p. 10). By our analysis, a structural cohesive device should describe an aspect of syntax in discourse. These items do not; therefore they should be excluded.

Finally, labeling ellipsis as a semantic cohesive device seems curious. Halliday and Hasan (1976) categorized ellipsis as a syntactic cohesive devise because it expresses a relationship between words or clauses. We wondered whether a different more expected result would be obtained using Halliday and Hasan's (1976) coding scheme rather than Ripich and Terrell's (1988). In this chapter, the categorization scheme of Halliday and Hasan was applied to explore further semantic and syntactic cohesion in the discourse of patients with Alzheimer's disease. In addition, we planned to undertake increasingly refined analysis of the coding categories of interest in order to distinguish cohesion patterns among and between patients with Alzheimer's disease and normals.

In the present study, the use of cohesive devices during open-ended conversation was examined in two moderately impaired Alzheimer's patients. The initial focus of our investigation was to explore those devices that are semantic in nature (lexical cohesion and reference) and those that are syntactic (substitution, ellipsis, and conjunction), to see if the use of each type of device by the Alzheimer's patients differs from that of nondemented subjects. Further analysis involved examining the subtypes within each of Halliday and Hasan's categories of cohesive devices.

DESCRIPTION OF CASES

Two mid-stage female bilingual[1] (English–Yiddish) patients with the diagnosis of probable Alzheimer's disease were studied. These patients (F.D. and M.E.) were part of a larger study on code switching in bilingual Alzheimer's disease (De Santi, Obler, Sabo-Abramson, & Goldberger, 1989). Two of the four subjects in that study were excluded here because their corpora supplied limited interactive conversational discourse: One patient talked very little, whereas the other patient talked excessively and the examiner produced primarily conversational maintainers, such as "mm-hum."

The diagnosis of Alzheimer's disease was determined by a medical gerontologist and was based on progression of impairment in memory, language, cognitive, and behavioral skills. The possibility that a pseudo-dementia accounted for the progression of symptoms was ruled out based on medical tests and medical history. The stage of Alzheimer's disease was determined by the degree of language impairment as described by Obler and Albert (1984). In particular, the language changes characteristic of Stages 3–4 include difficulty telling a coherent story and discourse characterized by press of speech that is devoid of meaning with paragrammatisms and clang associations. The AD patients were residents of a geriatric institute.[2] The neurologically normal subjects resided in communities on Long Island. Demographic information is presented in Table 12.1.

PROCEDURES

A complete description of the procedures used to obtain the language sample can be found in De Santi et al. (1989). For the purposes of this chapter, only the conversational portion of the English discourse of F.D and M.E. with S.D. (the examiner) and of M.E. with D.E. (her son) were analyzed. S.D. is a monolingual English speaker. D.E. has some working knowledge of Yiddish but is not fluent in that language. The discourse between the examiner and the Alzheimer's patients arose during the introductory portion of the testing sessions, during breaks between testing, and during the time rapport was being established. Both subjects conversed with the examiner (S.D.) and subject M.E. also conversed with her son, D.E. The discourse between M.E. and D.E. arose during a family visit that occurred when S.D. was also visiting M.E. The discourse sample consisted of 178 conversational turns for F.D. and 291 conversational turns for M.E. The discourse of the two neurologically normal subjects, D.E. and S.D.,

---

[1]There is no reason to believe the bilingualism influenced the use of cohesive devices, however, we cannot rule out any subtle influence.

[2]The authors wish to thank the Parker Jewish Geriatric Institute, New Hyde Park, New York, for their cooperation in this study.

TABLE 12.1
Demographic Information on Subjects

Subjects	*Age*	*Sex*	*L1*	*L2*	*Age L2*	*Ed.*	*Stage of Disease*
F.D.	89	F	English	Yiddish	0	Grade 12	1
M.E.	87	F	Yiddish	English	19	Grade 8	3–4
S.D.	30	F	English	None	n/a	PhD	Normal
D.E.	54	M	English	Yiddish	0	Master's	Normal

Note. L1 = First learned language
L2 = Second learned language

served as the control data.[3] Two hundred fifty-four conversational turns for S.D. with M.E., 180 conversational turns for S.D. with F.D., and 77 conversational turns for D.E. with M.E. were analyzed.

Discourse samples were transcribed orthographically, following a format that recorded each conversational turn on a separate line. A *conversational turn* was defined as a segment of speech initiated by one interlocutor that ended when the next interlocutor spoke. A turn could consist of a portion of a phrase, one or more phrases, or a conversational maintainer (e.g., "ah-hah"). Each conversational turn was numbered for each interlocutor in consecutive order, for example:

1S. Where were you born (F.D.)?
1F. I was born on the East Side.
2S. Oh, good, and uh
2F. I was a high school graduate. (1)

All verbalizations were transcribed, including interjections, unintelligible utterances, and the rare non-English utterances.

Words were coded for instances of appropriate cohesion only. Inappropriate cohesion occurred rarely in the data and was not analyzed (F.D. had 2 instances of inappropriate cohesion and M.E. had 12). Note that this rare occurrence contrasts with previous reports (Ehrlich, 1990; Ripich & Terrell, 1988). According to Halliday and Hasan (1976), a single instance of cohesion occurs whenever some word or construction can be interpreted only by referring to some other element in the text (written or spoken). In order for the cohesion to be appropriate, both the presupposing and the presupposed elements must be present and identifiable in the discourse, as in the following example where the use of "he" and "him" refers to M.E.'s son.

[3]Because the communicative interaction in which the Alzheimer's patient typically engages involves significantly younger individuals (e.g., medical staff or family members), age was not controlled or manipulated as an experimental variable.

S.D. "How is (son's name)?"
M.E. "*He*'s alright."
S.D. "Did *he* visit you?"
M.E. "I visit *him*." (2)

The coding scheme outlined by Halliday and Hasan (1976) to use in analyzing texts is multilayered, such that one can code to various levels of specificity. Because the analysis undertaken in this project was intended to determine whether the Alzheimer's patients show gross differences in their use of syntactic and semantic cohesive devices compared to that of neurologically normal individuals, much of the detail incorporated into this system was not adopted. In the initial analysis, only the five primary types of cohesion in English discussed by Halliday and Hasan were used to code the discourse. A definition and example of each of the five follows. In the example, cohesive devices are italicized and the code for that device is given.

Primary Types of Cohesion

Type 1: Reference. This first type of cohesion consists of any use of pronouns (R1), demonstratives (R2) including *here*, *there*, and *then* as well as the definite article, or comparative items (R3) including *more*, *less*, *another*, *similar* when preceded by a referent within the text. The defining feature of *reference* is a cohesive relation of identity. In other words, the referent remains constant.

S: What about your husband?
F: *He's* a wonderful man. (R1: pronominal reference) (3)

Type 2: Lexical Cohesion. Type 2 is essentially a reiteration or a restating of previous items said by oneself or one's conversational partner. The simplest type is exact repetition of a word (L1). Somewhat more complex is the use of synonym or homonym (L2), a superordinate (L3), a "general" item such as *thing* or *person* (L4), or collocation (L5), "the association of lexical items that regularly co-occur" (Halliday & Hasan, 1976, p. 284) for example, peanut butter and jelly.

S: Now first of all, um, you speak another language.
F: No, I don't *speak*—I *speak* Jewish. (L1: same word) (4)

Type 3: Substitution. Substitution involves replacing a noun phrase, verb phrase, or clause with another item. In English, there is a fairly small set of regular substituting items; *one* and *some* for nouns (S1), *do* for verbs (S2; this includes constructions such as *do that, do likewise*) and *so* and *not* for clauses (S3; such as *I don't think so*, when preceded by appropriate supporting context).

S: You like that?
F: I *do*, yeah. (S2: verbal substitution) (5)

Type 4: Ellipsis. Type 4 occurs when one must fill in some specific structural "slot" by referring to something else in the text. Usually, there is an omission of a noun phrase (E1), a verb phrase (E2), or a clause (E3).

S: How old were you when you when you first started to learn English?
F: I was 18. (E3: clausal ellipsis) (6)

Type 5: Conjunction. This final type of cohesion includes adverbial constructions as well as the usual set of coordinating conjunctions. The cohesion here is indirect because the conjunctive items do not refer to other elements as such, but rather their meanings presuppose other elements. Conjunctions are broken down according to the kind of relationship they express: additive (C1; *and, furthermore*); adversative (C2; *but, however*); causal (C3; *so, consequently*); temporal (C4; *then, meanwhile*); and continuative (C5; *now, well, anyway*).

S: Are you tired today?
M: *Well* of course I'm a little more tired. (C5: continuative conjunction) (7)

Substitution and ellipsis are considered to be relations between linguistic elements or structures. Although Halliday and Hasan regard conjunction as a separate category, we have included it with syntactic cohesive devices because conjunctions link phrases. These are thought of as grammatical relations rather than semantic ones and were categorized as types of syntactic cohesive devises. Lexical cohesion and reference were codified as semantic cohesive devices by Halliday and Hasan and for this analysis as well. (Recall that, by contrast, Ripich and Terrell coded reference, conjunction, and ellipsis to be examples of semantic cohesion.)

All transcripts were coded by a linguist. Reliability for coding was determined by a second linguist trained in the scheme, who recoded approximately 200 turns per subject. Agreement between the two linguists was $r = .90$ ($p < .001$). When discrepancies arose, the two linguists discussed the problem until a resolution was reached.

ANALYSES AND RESULTS

To examine our data using a paradigm similar to Ripich and Terrell (1988), we looked at cohesive devices according to overall linguistic level (semantic and syntactic). Due to the limited number of subjects no statistical procedures were

TABLE 12.2
Proportion of Semantic and Syntactic Cohesive Devices
(Per Total Number of Words)

	Alzheimer's Patients		*Control Subjects*	
Device	*M.E.*	*F.D.*	*S.D*	*D.E.*
Semantic	17%	19%	13%	13%
Syntactic	7%	7%	6%	5%

Note. Semantic cohesive devices include lexical cohesion and reference. Syntactic cohesive devices include ellipsis, conjunction, and substitution.

undertaken. Individual data are reported so the reader can view the range of each subject's behaviors. The percentages of the total number of words consisting of appropriate semantic and syntactic cohesive devices used by each subject are listed in Table 12.2. This proportion was obtained by dividing the number of occurrences of a device by the total number of words produced in the discourse sample.

Data analysis revealed that the Alzheimer's subjects used at least as many cohesive devices, regardless of type, as the normal control subjects, or even more. The finding that semantic cohesion occurred with slightly greater frequency in the Alzheimer's patients than in the normal controls is in direct conflict with the results of Ripich and Terrell (1988), who reported that their Alzheimer's group used less semantic cohesion than normals. Moreover, the literature on Alzheimer's disease in general leads us to expect evidence of semantic impairment (Bayles & Kaszniak, 1987; Obler & Albert, 1984), which we thought would be expressed through disruption in semantic cohesion. That semantic cohesion is problematic in the discourse of Alzheimer's disease could not be supported in the present investigation. Thus, it appears that cohesion may not be a critical indicator of semantic impairment because appropriate use of cohesive devices alone does not indicate that discourse will appear logical to the listener.

The fact that semantic cohesion occurred with somewhat greater frequency in the Alzheimer's group than in the normal controls warranted further investigation. We next examined the subtypes of cohesive devices that comprised the semantic and syntactic categories. The data are shown in Table 12.3.

By this analysis, the Alzheimer's group used at least as many cohesive devices as the control subjects for all subtypes with the possible exception of substitution. Looking at the data one can also see that lexical cohesion was the only subtype where both Alzheimer's subjects looked somewhat different from the control subjects. The Alzheimer's patients produced proportionally more lexical cohesion devices than did the controls. Lexical cohesion is a semantic cohesive device, thus the fact that it occurs with greater frequency in the Alzheimer's group is counter-intuitive. A more detailed analysis of lexical cohesion was undertaken by delineating the type of devices within this category (see Table 12.4).

TABLE 12.3
Types of Semantic and Syntactic Cohesive Devices
(Per Total Number of Words)

	Alzheimer's Patients		*Control Subjects*	
Device	*M.E.*	*F.D.*	*S.D*	*D.E.*
Lexical	14%	16%	10%	10%
Reference	4%	3%	3%	4%
Ellipses	6%	4%	3%	3%
Conjunction	2%	2%	2%	1%
Substitution	2%	5%	6%	7%

Note. Lexical cohesion = restatement of a previous item.
Reference = using pronouns, demonstratives, or comparative items.
Ellipsis = omission of noun phrase, verb phrase, or clause.
Conjunction = using adverbials or coordinating conjunctions.
Substitution = replacement of a noun phrase, verb phrase, or clause.

The most frequent type of lexical cohesion used by all speakers was repetition. The other subtypes of lexical cohesion, namely the use of synonym, superordinate, general items, and collocation occurred rarely, thus we did not examine them any further. The Alzheimer's subjects seem to use repetition far more frequently than the control subjects. We therefore examined it in greater detail.

For this analysis, repetitions were coded for their distance from the stimulus production. Repetitions that were four or fewer of a speaker's turns away from the stimulus were coded as near repetitions, whereas those that were greater than four turns away were distant repetitions. All repetitions were also coded as self-repetitions (speaker repeated something he or she said previously) or other repetitions (speaker repeated the other interlocutor's speech). Various examples occur in the following discourse sample (the repetition is italicized and the type is in parentheses).

M.E. "I had no sisters, just brothers. Boys, boys. The picture of Dorian Gray. From school we had the book. I just had sons and no girls."
S.D. "And what?"
M.E. "Three *sons*. (self-near repetition) Your mother's working?"
S.D. "Yep."
M.E. "So, that's the way the ball bounces."
S.D. "m-hum."
M.E. "I have an old *mother*." (self-near repetition)
S.D. "Do you?"
M.E. "She is in shoe business (laughs). Yeah, *shoes*. She bakes everyday. Bread, rolls. *Shoe business*, I forgot myself." (self-near repetitions)
S.D. "But you *forgot*. Did you work in her *shoe* place?" (other near repetitions)

TABLE 12.4
Types of Lexical Cohesive Devices

	Alzheimer's Patients		*Control Subjects*	
Device	*M.E.*	*F.D.*	*S.D*	*D.E.*
Repetition (L1)	11%	15%	8%	6%
Synonym (L2)	1%	0.2%	0.3%	0.9%
Superordinate (L3)	0.5%	0.1%	0%	0.3%
General Item (L4)	0.1%	0%	0%	0%
Collocation (L5)	1%	1%	1%	2%

M.E. "No I don't *work.*" (other-near repetition)
S.D. "Did you *work* before?" (other-near repetition)
M.E. "Nothing, nothing I don't *work.*" (other-near repetition)
S.D. "You never *worked*?" (other-near repetition)
M.E. "*Never worked.* (other-near repetition) Oh, how old am I, this to be afraid you *never worked.* (self-near repetition) My parents *work.* (self-near repetition) *Picture of Dorian Gray.*" (self-distant repetition) (8)

The proportions of repetitions that were categorized as near, distant, self, and other are displayed in Table 12.5.

These numbers show that all interlocutors display different styles in using repetitions. Patient M.E. frequently used repetitions that were near to the stimulus, produced by either of the two speakers. Patient F.D., on the other hand, used more near repetitions of stimulus words that were initially produced by the interlocutor. In conversation with patient M.E., control S.D. appeared to mirror the patient's style by frequently using near repetitions of stimuli initially used by either herself or M.E. When S.D. conversed with patient F.D., a different

TABLE 12.5
Types of Repetitions

Device	*M.E.*	*F.D.*	*S.D. with M.E.*	*S.D. with F.D.*	*D.E.*
Self-near	38%	19%	47%	28%	66%
Self-distant	26%	34%	12%	20%	15%
Other-near	35%	44%	39%	34%	15%
Other-distant	1%	2%	3%	18%	3%

Note. Self-near = repeating an item speaker said during the past four turns.
Self-distant = repeating an item speaker said that is more than four turns away.
Other-near = repeating an item that the interlocutor said during past four turns.
Other-distant = repeating an item spoken by the interlocutor which is more than four turns away.

style emerged: Although all types of repetitions occurred, near repetitions of items initially generated by F.D. were most frequent. Control D.E., by contrast, produced more near repetitions of stimuli that had been said by himself (i.e., D.E. did not adopt the patient's style). In summary, this analysis showed that a variety of repetition styles emerge during conversation. As control S.D.'s data showed, one's style may change with different conversational partners.

The high occurrence of near repetitions in the discourse of all subjects interested us and we examined them in greater detail. First, we looked at other-near repetitions for each of the four subjects following a coding system for contingent utterances in order to determine if this much-used category reflected individual differences. Contingent utterances, according to Frome-Loeb and Schwartz (1990), are adjacent to another speaker's utterance and related to it by topic, structure, or content. We coded an other-near repetition as *borrowing*, when the speaker used a portion or all of the interlocutor's utterance adding some unique words (Clark, 1974); *imitative*, when the speaker reproduced all or part of the interlocutor's speech without adding any new words; or *content-related*, when the speaker used just one content word from the preceding discourse (see Table 12.6).

Most of patient F.D.'s other-near repetitions (58%) were borrowed. That is, F.D. tended to use the same syntactic frame as the interlocutor. For example, when asked "Were they (her parents) born in this country?", D.F. responded "They were born in this country, yes." This response gave the impression that D.F.'s language was far more sophisticated than, we suspect, it really was. D.F.'s second most frequently used strategy was imitative repetitions (23%) in which she repeated exactly what the interlocutor said. The rarest type of repetition was content-related repetitions (19%).

Patient M.E. had a different conversational style. The most common type of repetition she used was content related (66%). M.E. basically used the same proportion of imitation (16%) and borrowing (17%). Although she produced many utterances that were appropriate content-related repetitions (S.D. "What about your *mother*?" M.E. "No, my *mother* is gone for many years."), some

TABLE 12.6
Types of Other-Near Repetitions

Device	*M.E.*	*F.D.*	*S.D. with M.E.*	*S.D. with F.D.*	*D.E.*
Borrowing	17%	58%	17%	10%	20%
Imitative	16%	23%	13%	0%	20%
Content-related	66%	19%	70%	90%	60%

Note. Borrowing = speaker used portion of all of interlocutor's utterance adding some unique words.

Imitative = speaker produced all or part of interlocutor's utterance without adding any new words.

Content related = speaker used just one content word from the preceding discourse.

routines (overlearned phrases) were generated from a word the interlocutor produced. For example, when asked "Do you remember my name?", M.E. responded "Thy name is woman." Subsequently M.E. used this phrase often after the interlocutor said the word "name."

S.D., the examiner, had a style that was similar to M.E. in that content-related repetitions were most frequent (90% in conversation with F.D. and 70% in conversation with M.E.). Borrowing occurred with a frequency of 17% when S.D. was in conversation with M.E. and 10% with F.D. Imitative repetitions only occurred with M.E. (13%). Other-near repetitions were relatively infrequent in the speech of D.E., a control subject. Of the other-near repetitions produced, 60% were content related, 20% were borrowing, and 20% were imitative. In summary, this analysis reinforced the notion that different communicative styles were exhibited by the different speakers.

The last examination we undertook was of self-near repetitions (the repeated portion was from the speaker's previous utterance), to see if communicative styles of the speakers were as diverse when using a different type of repetition. We coded these repetitions using essentially the system described for other-near repetitions but with one additional category. In addition to borrowing, imitative, and content-related repetitions, we coded for *routines*, that is, rote phrases generated by the speaker. This category was added because none of the other categories adequately captured a speaker's idiosyncratic phrase production. For example, S.D. would often say, "Oh, that's nice" when commenting about something the interlocutor said.

At noted in Table 12.7, 38% of patient F.D.'s self-near repetitions were coded as borrowing. Imitations (21%), routines (21%), and content-related repetitions (20%) were basically undistinguishable from each other. This pattern is similar to that produced by this subject for other-near repetitions where borrowing was the most used repetition type.

TABLE 12.7
Types of Self-Near Repetitions

Device	*M.E.*	*F.D.*	*S.D. with M.E.*	*S.D. with F.D.*	*D.E.*
Borrowing	0%	38%	7%	8%	0%
Imitative	6%	21%	0%	0%	9%
Content-related	67%	20%	83%	77%	77%
Routines	23%	21%	10%	15%	14%

Note. Borrowing = speaker used portion of all of interlocutor's utterance adding some unique words.

Imitative = speaker produced all or part of interlocutor's utterance without adding any new words.

Content related = speaker used just one content word from the preceding discourse.

Routines = speaker generated a rote phrase from a word the interlocutor produced.

Patient M.E. did not produce the same pattern of self-near repetitions as other-near repetitions. Although content-related repetitions remained this subject's most frequently used repetition type (67%), borrowing was not used at all. Instead M.E.'s repetitions were routines (23%) or imitations (6%).

For self-near repetitions, control S.D. used mostly content-related repetitions (77% with F.D., 83% with M.E.). Routines were the next most used (15% with F.D and 10% with M.E.) and borrowing the least used (8% with F.D. and 7% with M.E.). D.E., the other control, also used content-related repetitions most frequently (77%), followed by routines (14%) and then imitations (9%).

The subcategorization of repetition into types indicates that speakers used different subtypes of other- and near-repetitions within a conversation. Through this analysis one also sees each speaker's idiosyncratic speech style as indicated by the amount of routines and imitations produced.

CONCLUSIONS

This project examined cohesive devices in the conversational discourse of two Alzheimer's patients in the moderate stage of the disease. Discourse was examined for both semantic and syntactic cohesive devices. Because AD affects the semantic system, we expected that there would be a reduction in the use of those cohesive devices categorized as semantic. To our surprise, we did not find this to be the case. In fact, semantic cohesive devices, namely lexical cohesion, were produced frequently by the two Alzheimer's patients, as they were by the normals. We must conclude that, as Ripich and Terrell (1988) reported, cohesion, and more specifically semantic cohesion, is a poor indicator of semantic impairment in the language of Alzheimer's disease.

To understand this finding, lexical cohesion was examined in detail. It was discovered that repetitions occurred more frequently than other devices for both patients and controls. Although the more general analyses had not distinguished between subjects, a more refined analysis of repetition revealed differences between the two patients. M.E. tended to use content-related repetitions where one word from the previous discourse unit was repeated and the rest of the utterance was produced on-line. M.E. also used many routines which appeared to serve as conversational fillers and did not add information to the conversation. F.D., on the other hand, tended to borrow a portion of the preceding discourse from the interlocutor and to generate little of her own on-line conversation.

The fact that F.D. was able to use the preceding discourse as a way of framing and maintaining conversational discourse provided her with an important linguistic strategy. In contrast, M.E. used a topic-related repetition strategy to maintain conversation. In terms of quality of conversational discourse, using this more detailed cohesive device analysis, M.E. appears to have more conversational skills preserved despite the fact that by the staging system used, her dementia was somewhat more advanced than F.D.'s. The repetition of a topic-related word meant that M.E. had to generate more of the discourse than F.D., who used more of the interlocutor's speech to produce discourse.

Not only did the two Alzheimer's patients clearly have different conversational styles, the control S.D. also showed varied styles depending on her conversational partner. S.D.'s conversational style was essentially similiar to the patient M.E., in that the rank order and relative percentage of repetition types were the same in their conversation. When S.D. was conversing with F.D., a different pattern was found. Not only was the rank order of repetition types different between the control and F.D., but the occurrence of certain types of repetitions (e.g., other-distant) was greater. The variability of the control's speech was probably reflective of the style each conversational partner presented.

We must consider the findings of Ripich and Terrell (1988), to represent a good first approximation of those presented here. Although our study is limited in the number of subjects evaluated (recall, however, that control subjects were younger than the Alzheimer's group), group differences in conversational discourse still emerged. There are distinct cohesion-related discourse strategies used during conversation by both Alzheimer's patients and normals (and, indeed, by a given normal in conversation with different Alzheimer's patients).

Moreover, we believe that repetitions during discourse might serve a strategic purpose and should be examined further in the language of Alzheimer's disease. For example, Bayles et al. (1985) showed increased perseveration by patients with Alzheimer's disease (relative to controls) who were describing objects. Our finding leads us to expect that analyzing these responses in depth could produce a more informative picture of perseveration. Because there is variability in discourse performance, that is, the use of repetitions across subjects (M.E. vs. F.D.) and within subjects (S.D.), the study presented here should be replicated using a larger number of patients with Alzheimer's disease with age-matched controls.

We conclude that word or phrase repetition, and the role it plays in language, is important in the study of language in Alzheimer's disease. Perseveration, palilalia, and echolalia are types of repetition associated with Alzheimer's disease that have been attributed to nonlinguistic deficits (Hier et al., 1985). *Perseveration*, defined as the inappropriate repetition of an entire phrase (Hier et al., 1985), has been regarded as a reflection of difficulties changing mental set. These authors also found that perseveration correlated with anomia, and suggested that it might indicate a semantic accessing problem associated with Alzheimer's disease. The analysis presented in this chapter, by contrast, suggests that repetitions may provide important linguistic strategies—necessary, perhaps, when more general semantic problems interfere with linguistic abilities.

It is possible that the repetition in discourse changes characteristically throughout the course of Alzheimer's disease. The data reported on here lead us to speculate that early in the disease, topic-related repetitions occur most frequently, whereas use of routines (i.e. formulaic utterances) is limited. As the disease progresses, one might expect a decrease in topic-related repetitions and an increase in borrowing, imitations, and routines. In advanced Alzheimer's disease, it seems likely that routines will become the most frequent type of repetition with the prevalence of other types decreasing and eventually being lost.

REFERENCES

Bayles, K. (1982). Language function in senile dementia. *Brain and Language, 16*, 265–280.

Bayles, K. (1985). Communication in dementia. In H. Ulatowska (Ed.), *The aging brain: Communication in the elderly*. Boston: College Hill Press.

Bayles, K., & Kaszniak, A. (1987). *Communication and cognition in normal aging and dementia*. Boston: College Hill Press.

Bayles, K., Tomoeda, C., & Caffrey, J. (1982). Language and dementia producing diseases. *Communicative Disorders, 10*, 131–146.

Bayles, K., Tomoeda, C., Kaszniak, A., Stern, L., & Eagans, K. (1985). Verbal perseveration of dementia patients. *Brain and Language, 25*, 102–116.

Clark, R. (1974). Performing without competence. *Journal of Child Language, 4*, 1–10.

De Santi, S., Obler, L. K., Sabo-Abramson, H., & Goldberger, J. (1989). Discourse abilities and deficits in multilingual dementia. In H. Brownell & Y. Joanette (Eds.), *Discourse ability and brain damage: Theoretical and empirical perspectives* (pp. 224–233). New York: Springer-Verlag.

Ehrlich, J. (1990). *The influence of structure on the content of oral narrative in adults with dementia of the Alzheimer's type*. Unpublished doctoral dissertation, CUNY, New York.

Frome-Loeb, D., & Schwartz, R. (1990). Language characteristics of a linguistically precocious child. *First Language, 10*, 1–18.

Halliday, M., & Hasan, R. (1976). *Cohesion in English*. London: Longmans.

Hamilton, H. (in press). *Conversations with an Alzheimer's patient*. Cambridge: Cambridge University Press.

Hier, D., Hagenlocker, K., & Shindler, A. (1985). Language disintegration in dementia on a picture description task. *Brain and Language, 25*, 117–133.

Nicholas, M., Obler, L. K., Albert, M., & Helm-Estabrooks, N. (1985). Empty speech in Alzheimer's disease and fluent aphasia. *Journal of Speech and Hearing Research, 38*, 405–410.

Obler, L. K., & Albert, M. (1984). Language in aging. In M. Albert (Ed.), *Clinical neurology of aging* (pp.). New York: Oxford University Press.

Ripich, D., & Terrell, B. (1988). Patterns of discourse cohesion and coherence in Alzheimer's disease. *Journal of Speech and Hearing Disorders, 53*, 8–15.

Ripich, D., Vertes, D., Whitehouse, P., Fulton, S., & Ekelman, B. (1991). Turn-taking and speech act patterns in the discourse of senile dementia of the Alzheimer's type patients. *Brain and Language, 40*, 330–343.

Chapter 13

Communication Patterns in End-Stage Alzheimer's Disease: Pragmatic Analyses

Mary Anne Causino Lamar
Christchurch, New Zealand

Loraine K. Obler
The City University of New York Graduate School

Janice E. Knoefel
Martin L. Albert
Boston University School of Medicine and
Boston Veterans Administration Medical Center

Little is known about communication in end-stage Alzheimer's disease. Obler and Albert (1984) reported that individuals lose the press of speech that is characteristic of earlier stages and are often mute. Palilalia and clang associations are common in the limited speech that is produced, and comprehension appears to be extremely impaired. There are reports, however, that alongside this severe impairment, individuals may retain some ability to communicate. Obler (1981) noted some ability to interpret intonation patterns. Schwartz, Marin, and Saffran (1979) reported some effective use of gestural communication. De Ajuriaguerra and Tissot (1975) observed some sensitivity to eye contact and appropriate use of extralinguistic context in both comprehension and production. Bayles, Tomoeda, and Caffrey (1982) noted preservation of "automatic language associated with commonly encountered situations" (p. 136). Preliminary results from Bayles, Kaszniak, and Tomoeda's (1987) study of structured conversational interaction in late-stage Alzheimer's patients indicated that a number of conversational skills are still available to at least some patients. These include maintenance of eye contact during conversation, correction of semantically incorrect statements made by the conversational partner, production of relevant responses to compliments and statements of thanks, providing certain kinds of clarification upon request, responding appropriately when offered a handshake, and others.

To our knowledge, this study is the first systematic investigation of communication in an even later stage of Alzheimer's disease, which we refer to as the *end stage*. The focus of this investigation is the pragmatic aspect of communication. The term *pragmatics* is used here to refer to conventions governing the use of language in context and the intentions expressed through communication. The specific aspects of pragmatics we considered are outlined in the appendix.

Many investigations of pragmatics in individuals with communicative disorders have emphasized pragmatic deficits. Rather than searching only for deficits, we looked also for aspects of pragmatics that are preserved and the contexts in which they occur. Albert (1980) recommended that researchers and clinicians look for "signs of strength" in addition to "signs of deterioration" in the elderly in order that new therapies can be developed based on these "pockets of strength" (p. 145).

The primary procedure for carrying out this investigation was modified naturalistic observation, a procedure whereby subjects are observed in on-going social interaction in their natural environment, in this case, as they go about their daily routines. Naturalistic observation was selected for three major reasons. First, this procedure has been used successfully in studies of pragmatics with other brain-injured adults. According to Davis and Wilcox (1985), "Of all pragmatic procedures, natural observations yield the most representative information and, as such, are probably the most useful for planning and conducting treatment" (p. 83). Holland (1982), in her study of functional communication in aphasic adults, noted that this method is particularly useful for clinical research because it allows one to observe important contextual parameters, the patient's overall communicativeness, and specific communicative strategies that are successful as well as ones that are unsuccessful.

Second, use of naturalistic observation is especially important as a method of studying communication patterns in the end stage of Alzheimer's because it allows these severely impaired individuals to be studied in a familiar environment where they may be expected to have the most communicative success. De Ajuriaguerra and Tissot (1975), in their study of language degeneration in dementia, noted that in a "natural, practical linguistic and extralinguistic situation" (p. 332), individuals produced and comprehended material that they had been unable to produce or comprehend in "artificial, purely linguistic situations" (p. 332).

Third, naturalistic observation is widely recognized by social scientists (Cairns & Green, 1979; Manheim & Simon, 1977; Parke, 1979; Yarrow & Waxler, 1979) as particularly important in the exploratory stage of research because, unlike the other procedures listed previously, it does not exclude potentially relevant aspects of the context. Parke (1979) recommended further that naturalistic field observation be employed when there is little or no background on a topic in order to provide the basis for generating hypotheses that can later be tested more rigorously in an experimental design.

We modified strict naturalistic observation procedures in two ways. First, a researcher was always visibly present in the room with the subjects. Second, deliberately, in half of the conversations with each subject, it was the investigator who was the subject's conversational partner.

Most investigations of pragmatics examine a small set of behaviors (Duchan, 1984). Because of its exploratory nature, however, this study surveys a broad range of behaviors (68 different aspects of pragmatics, grouped into 13 major parameters) in order to determine which of these warrant more in-depth exploration in subsequent studies.

The specific research questions addressed in the current study are: What pragmatic behaviors are spared in the end stage of Alzheimer's? Are there distinct subgroups within this population on the basis of pragmatic performance?

METHOD

Subjects

Ten patients with a diagnosis of probable Alzheimer's disease in the end stage, all residents of the same chronic care hospital, served as subjects. The diagnosis of Alzheimer's was based on the following criteria (McKhann et al., 1984):

1. progressive decline (as reported through case history) and deficits (as identified by examination) in at least three of the following five areas—memory, language, visuospatial abilities, higher cognitive functions, affect/behavior;
2. no history of alcoholism, serious psychiatric disease, or severe head trauma;
3. a score of 4 or less on the Hachinski Scale (Hachinski, 1983), a scale used in diagnosis of multi-infarct dementia;
4. negative laboratory tests (including CAT scan of head, lumbar puncture, urinalysis, blood screen [18 factor], vitamin B12 and folate level; and thyroid function tests);
5. no disturbance of consciousness;
6. onset between ages 40 and 90; and
7. absence of systemic disorders or other brain diseases that in and of themselves could account for the progressive deficits in memory and cognition.

In addition, criteria for identifying the end stage of Alzheimer's consisted of the following:

1. a score of less than 25 (out of 144) on the Mattis Dementia Rating Scale (Mattis, 1976); and
2. a score of less than 50 (out of 105) on the Barthel Scale of Activities of Daily Living (Mahoney & Barthel, 1965).

Seventeen potential subjects were originally selected on the basis of behavioral patterns and medical history. Consent for participation in the study was obtained from the legal guardians of 16. Of these, 3 were excluded for scoring above 25 on the Mattis Dementia Rating Scale, 1 was excluded because of unstable medical condition, and 2 died before data collection was complete.

Table 13.1 presents background information for the 10 remaining subjects. Their ages ranged from 70 to 89 years ($M = 81.6$ years; $SD = 6.5$ years). Nine subjects were female and 1 was male; 3 were African American and 7 were White. Handedness information was available for only 7 of the 10 subjects; of those 7, all were right-handed. The years since onset for each subject were measured from the time the individual's family first noted behavior changes characteristic of Alzheimer's disease. This time period ranged from 2 to 14 years ($M = 5.8$ years; $SD = 3.5$ years). All subjects were native speakers of English, 8 of whom were born in the United States, 1 in Canada, and 1 in Barbados.

Data Collection

Discourse samples were obtained from four 15-minute conversations with each subject. Two of the four conversations were held with a familiar member of the hospital staff who was identified by the head nurse on that ward as being the caregiver most successful in communicating with that subject. Two other conversations were held with the investigator. All conversations were held in locations very familiar to the subjects (such as their own room or the recreation or dining room on their ward). Several of the conversations took place while the subjects were engaged in daily routines, such as eating, dressing, or washing. Each setting was selected according to reports from family and staff identifying the subjects' most communicative situations. Conversations concerned activities subjects were

TABLE 13.1
Characteristics of Subjects

*Subject**	*Age*	*Sex*	*Race*	*Handedness*	*Years Since Onset*
B.D.	78	F	African American	Right	3
I.E.	82	F	White	Right	5
N.E.	70	F	White	Right	6
I.N.	82	M	White	Right	2
H.N.	78	F	White	Right	7
J.N.	89	F	White	—	7
K.O.	75	F	African American	—	—
I.W.	89	F	White	Right	4
H.Z.	84	F	White	Right	14
N.Z.	89	F	African American	—	4

*To protect the subjects' privacy, the initials used in this table and throughout the study are not the subjects' true initials.

immediately engaged in, the immediate environment, the subjects' family, hobbies, work experience, or other topics raised by the subjects themselves. No attempt was made to elicit specific pragmatic behaviors. Each conversation was started with a simple explanation of the purpose of the visit. Whenever a subject objected to participating in conversation or did not respond within the first 5 minutes, the conversation was postponed until a later time or date.

All conversations were audio-recorded using a Marantz PM 7450-5316 cassette recorder and a Sony ECM-210S Electret Condenser omni-directional microphone. Pertinent visual aspects of the context were recorded in writing.

Data Coding

Each conversation was transcribed, and 25 consecutive "turns" from each subject were selected for analysis. A "subject's turn" was defined operationally as one of the following: (a) one or more consecutive utterances, gestures, or communicative facial expressions by a subject including an unfilled pause of no more than 5 seconds; or (b) an interval of 3 to 30 seconds between two of the conversational partner's utterances during which the subject is expected (by the partner) to communicate but does not. Because we sought to identify those pragmatic behaviors subjects are capable of (rather than those that are typical of their conversation), the segment selected for analysis was one that included each subject's most responsive portions of the conversation.

Next, each of the 25 turns for each subject was assigned one of the following four ratings for any of the applicable 13 pragmatic parameters presented in Table 13.2. (A working definition of each of the 13 pragmatic parameters and a taxonomy of specific behaviors comprising these parameters is shown in the appendix.) This rating system was derived from a model proposed by Prutting and Kirchner (1983).

TABLE 13.2
Major Pragmatic Parameters

I. Protocol of discourse
 A. Control of topic
 B. Turns
 C. Feedback to conversational partner
 D. Presuppositions
 E. Requesting repairs
 F. Making repairs
 G. Social lubricants
II. Functions of discourse
 H. Directives
 I. Responses to directives
 J. Comments and representatives
 K. Acknowledging comments
 L. Expressives
 M. Commissives

Positive
1. Occurred appropriately

Negative
2. Occurred inappropriately
3. Did not occur when obligatory
4. Did not occur when likely

A hierarchy of spared pragmatic parameters was then established using the procedures described next. First, one of the following four summary descriptors was assigned to each pragmatic parameter for each subject:

1. Relatively spared: A given parameter was observed at least four times for a given subject, and at least 75% of these observations received a positive rating (i.e., occurred appropriately).
2. Variable: A given parameter was observed at least four times for a given subject, and fewer than 75% but at least 25% of these observations received a positive rating.
3. Severely impaired: A given parameter was observed at least four times for a given subject, and fewer than 25% of these observations received a positive rating.
4. Inconclusive: A given parameter was observed fewer than four times for a given subject.

Each of the 13 pragmatic parameters was then assigned a group summary descriptor based on the distribution of individual descriptors. The criteria for assigning group descriptors are listed here:

1. Relatively spared: At least half of the 10 subjects had a conclusive individual summary descriptor; and, of these subjects, the majority received the individual summary descriptor, relatively spared.
2. Variable: At least half of the 10 subjects had a conclusive individual summary descriptor; and, of these subjects, the majority received the individual summary descriptor, variable.
3. Severely impaired: At least half of the 10 subjects had a conclusive individual summary descriptor; and, of these subjects, the majority received the individual summary descriptor, severely impaired.
4. Mixed/Inconclusive:

At least half of the 10 subjects had a conclusive individual summary descriptor; however, of these subjects, no single individual summary descriptor was received by a majority.

Fewer than half of the 10 subjects had a conclusive summary descriptor.

Note that Levels 1–3 just given comprise a natural hierarchy, whereas Level 4 consists of categories that could not be placed within this hierarchy on the basis of available data.

RESULTS

Figure 13.1 shows the individual summary descriptor obtained by each subject across each of the 13 pragmatic parameters. Table 13.3 shows the resulting hierarchy of pragmatic behavior. As indicated in Table 13.3, four parameters—control of topic, turns, presuppositions, and directives—were spared for a majority of the subjects.

Control of topic was spared for 6 subjects and variable for the other 4. Most (86%) of the positive ratings for this parameter were assigned for the presence of a discernible topic (46%) and for continuation of the partner's topic (40%). Note that within this study a topic was considered discernible not necessarily on the basis of a single turn, but often on the basis of its context (linguistic or nonlinguistic). In fact, only 15% of the positive ratings for this aspect of topic pertained to turns in which the topic was specified verbally within that turn; 65% consisted of single, noncontent words, such as, "yes," "no," "okay," and "uh-huh." The remaining 20% were longer, elliptical utterances, such as "I don't want to," for which the topic was specified elsewhere in the context, usually by the interlocutor.

Another parameter, turns, was relatively spared for 7 subjects and variable for 3. Positive ratings were divided almost evenly between each of two aspects of turns considered here—length and latency. The ratio of positive to negative ratings for length of turns was approximately 6:1. Although one-word responses were common, more common than one would normally expect in conversation, this brevity was often appropriate, as the interlocutors tended to provide a supportive structure that allowed for such responses.

For latency of turns, the ratio of positive to negative ratings was approximately 4:1, with all negative ratings resulting from an excessively long latency (more than 3 seconds). There is reason to speculate, however, that the number of turns with excessively long latency would have been higher had the conversational partner not perceived the latency as a failure to respond and taken another turn.[1] The amount of time allotted by partners for subjects to respond was often shorter than the latencies subjects demonstrated (4 to 15 seconds) when given additional time. Furthermore, 2 subjects occasionally responded to questions and comments several turns after they occurred.[2]

[1]Garvey and Berninger (1981) reported that, in English, a pause of greater than 1 second normally signals the speaker's intent to transfer the speaking floor. Our subjects often required latencies as long as 30 seconds before responding.

[2]This practice, which Coulthard (1977) called *skip-connecting*, was observed by Hutchinson and Jensen (1980) at an earlier stage of dementia.

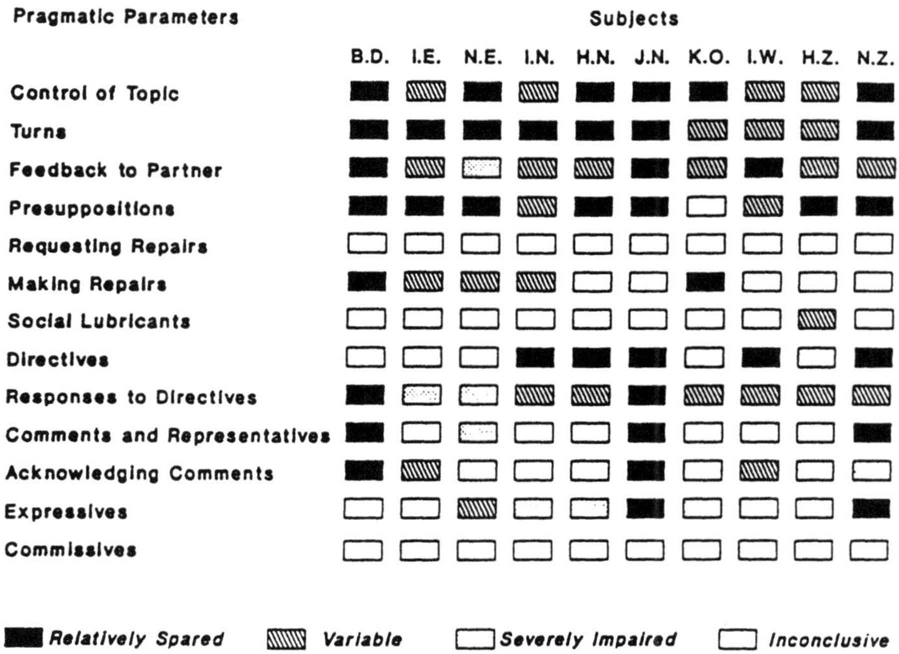

FIG. 13.1. Distribution of individual summary descriptors.

TABLE 13.3
Hierarchy of Spared Pragmatic Parameters for the Subjects as a Group

First Hierarchical Level: Relatively Spared
- Control of Topic
- Turns
- Presuppositions
- Directives

Second Hierarchical Level: Variable
- Feedback to Conversational Partner
- Response to Directives

Third Hierarchical Level: Severely Impaired
- Making Repairs

Mixed or Inconclusive Pragmatic Categories
- Acknowledging Comments
- Requesting Repairs
- Social Lubricants
- Comments and Representatives
- Expressives
- Commissives

A third parameter, presuppositions, was relatively spared for 7 subjects, variable for 2, and inconclusive for 1. At first glance, this strong performance for presuppositions is surprising, given the cognitive demands of shifting perspective, assessing the listener's knowledge, and monitoring the linguistic and nonlinguistic context, which are among the skills usually required for formulating appropriate presuppositions. Examination of the specific behaviors observed, however, will explain the high proportion of positive ratings. Of the 176 positive ratings accumulated by the group for presuppositions, 36% pertained to informativeness. Most (64%) of the turns receiving a positive rating for informativeness consisted of giving a yes–no response in the appropriate situation. Others consisted of simple gestures, such as tipping one's bowl toward the conversational partner when asked, "What are you eating?". Although such responses were appropriately informative, their presuppositional demands were slight.

Another aspect of presuppositions with a significant portion of the positive ratings (19%) is use of deixis. Most of these observations concerned use of deictic pronouns, such as "I," "you," "me," and "us," rather than other common deictic terms, such as adverbs of time or location or verbs, such as "come," "go," "give," or "take."

One other aspect of presuppositions, appreciation of physical context, also received a large portion of the positive ratings (19%). Among the observations of appropriate appreciation of physical context were: (a) beckoning to someone across the room, (b) raising one's voice when speaking to someone at a distance, and (c) commenting on a change in the environment (e.g., "It's getting dark."). The other two behaviors comprising presuppositions—cohesion and marking new and old information—earned, respectively, 13% and 10% of the positive ratings.

One additional parameter, directives, was spared for at least half the subjects. Most (51%) of the positive ratings for this parameter concerned expression of personal need or desire, such as, "I wanna talk to you," or requests for information, such as "What do you want?". Imperatives and requests for action also earned substantial portions of the positive ratings (18% and 13% respectively). Among the 10 subjects, there were only two negative ratings for directives (one for production of a directive when another speech act was required, another for a directive addressed to an absent addressee). The paucity of negative ratings may be largely an artifact of the scoring procedures used here (and, perhaps, intrinsic to assessment of certain speech acts); that is, seldom can it be said that production of certain speech acts (such as directives or commissives) is obligatory.

Other pragmatic parameters were appropriate less often than those just discussed, but were still within the repertoire of some subjects. Subjects inconsistently gave feedback to the conversational partner. Forms of appropriate feedback ranged from spontaneous correction of semantic information to turning one's head toward the speaker. Most (88%) of the negative ratings resulted from failure to give any feedback. Appropriate responses to directives included performance of requested actions, protesting, refusing, providing requested information, and transferring objects. Examples include complete verbal responses (such as, "Go ahead," when asked, "Do you mind if I sit down?"), a change in one's pattern of palilalia, a brief (2- to 3-second) break from wailing, and a shift in the direction of eye gaze.

The parameter, making repairs, was spared for only 2 of the 10 subjects, but 5 subjects did make at least one repair. Appropriate repairs usually took the form of repetition, elaboration, and increase in loudness. Lexical change, confirmation, specification, pitch change, and stress change were also noted at least once. Thus, a variety of repair strategies was available to the subjects as a group, but was not used consistently.

Results for other parameters were inconclusive (i.e., there were fewer than four observations per subject for more than half of the 10 subjects). These parameters included requesting repairs, comments and representatives, expressives, commissives, and social lubricants. It was observed during prescreening of subjects that some social lubricants, such as greetings, closings, and thanks tended to be within the repertoire of even the most impaired subjects. Because opportunities for expressing social lubricants tended to occur fewer than four times in the 25-turn samples analyzed here, conclusive summary descriptors could not be assigned.

Subject Subgroups

In order to identify subgroups among the subjects on the basis of pragmatic behavior, an agglomerative cluster analysis (Milligan, 1980) was performed. Only the four parameters with conclusive descriptors for all 10 subjects (control of topic, turns, feedback to conversational partner, and responses to directives) were included in the analysis.

Results showed three distinct patterns of performance, representing two subgroups and one individual with an idiosyncratic pattern. Figure 13.2 shows the average percentage of positive observations for each of the two subgroups across the four selected categories. Subgroup 1 consists of four subjects (B.D., H.N., J.N., and N.Z.) with relatively high scores for each of the four parameters considered here. Subgroup 2 consists of five subjects (I.E., N.E., I.N., K.O., and H.Z.) with a split pattern of high scores for topic control and turn-taking (i.e., latency and length of turns), but low scores for parameters that are indices of responsiveness.

The idiosyncratic pattern of the remaining subject is almost the mirror image of the pattern demonstrated by the subjects in Subgroup 2. This subject (I.W.) earned low scores for topic control and turns, but high scores for parameters that are indices of responsiveness. Subject I.W.'s communicative style differed from that of the other subjects in that she responded frequently, but most of her responses were judged inappropriate with regard to topic control and presuppositions.

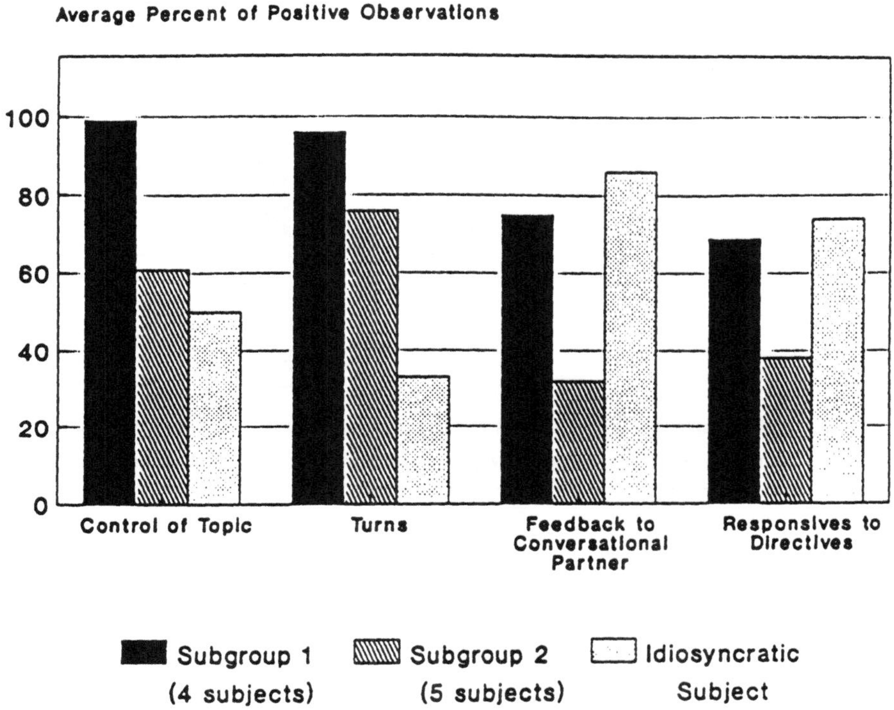

FIG. 13.2. Results of cluster analysis.

Figures 13.3 and 13.4 show the individual communicative profile of a representative subject from Subgroup 1 and from Subgroup 2, respectively.

DISCUSSION

Conclusions

A small set of pragmatic behaviors was spared for the subjects as a group and a larger set was within the repertoire of at least some of the subjects. The preservation of these aspects of pragmatics depended on the nondemented conversational partner bearing the weight of the conversation. Subjects seldom initiated conversation or were responsible for prolonging it. Obtaining responses from subjects often required that they be given a much longer time for responding than is ordinarily allowed in conversation. Messages frequently needed to be repeated, and subjects often needed an alerting signal, such as a tap on the shoulder, having their hand held, or being called by name, before they would respond. Under these extremely restricted conditions, the subjects as a group demonstrated a wide range of inconsistently appropriate pragmatic behaviors.

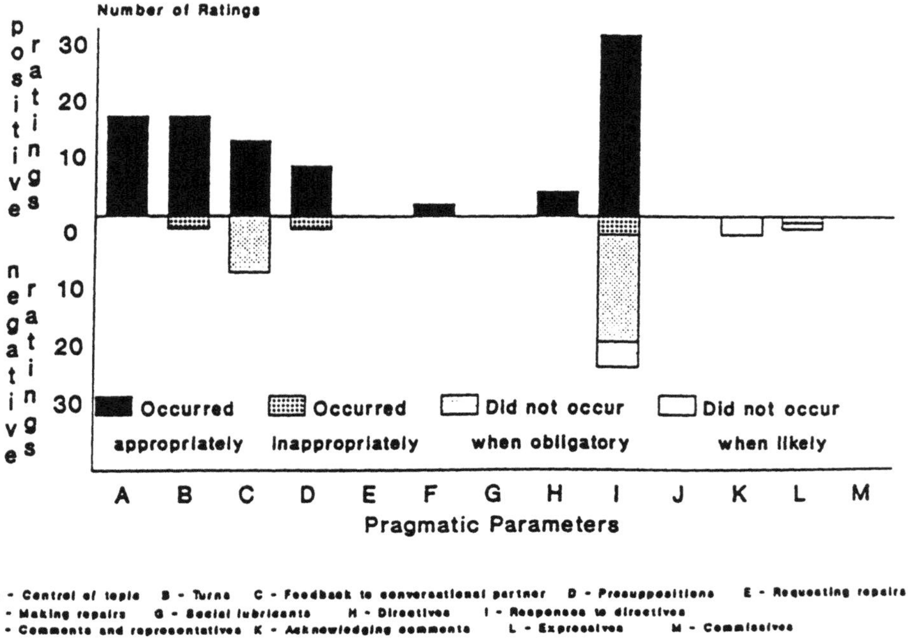

FIG. 13.3 Pragmatic profile of Subject H.N.

Among the pragmatic behaviors generally available to the subjects were several aspects of the protocol of conversation. Subjects were usually able to give a relevant response concerning a topic introduced by the conversational partner, to make appropriately informative contributions to the conversation, and to take turns of the appropriate length when their role was limited to giving highly elliptical responses to familiar questions. As the discourse demands increased, performance deteriorated and subjects' contributions tended to be irrelevant, incoherent, or absent.

Other aspects of the protocol of conversation, although more severely impaired than those previously discussed, were still available to some subjects. Most subjects inconsistently gave feedback to their conversational partner. Another critical element of conversation, requesting repairs, never occurred within the 25-turn samples, but occasionally, if requested, some subjects did attempt to make repairs.

It is more difficult to draw conclusions from the second pragmatic division investigated in this study, the functions of discourse. Of the six parameters comprising this division, only one, responses to directives, was observed frequently enough to draw conclusions for all 10 subjects. To some extent, this

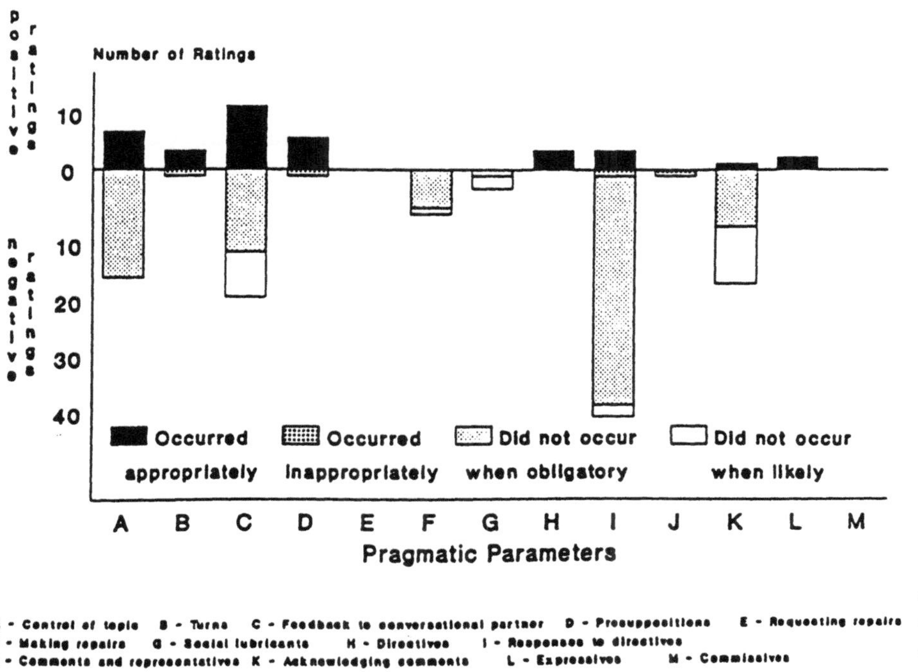

FIG. 13.4. Pragmatic profile of Subject I.E.

sparseness of data reflects a tendency on the part of the subjects not to initiate communication. That is, most subjects would respond to questions and imperatives (although these may require several repetitions, calling the subject's name, touching her or his shoulder, increasing loudness or other attention-arousing strategies), but would not comment spontaneously, express their feelings, or make a request.

Clinical Implications

It has been widely recognized that appropriate changes in the communicative context can lead to improved communication for individuals with dementia (Bayles et al., 1982, 1987; Lubinski, 1981; Ostuni & Santo Pietro, 1987; Tonkovich, 1984). The patterns of spared and impaired pragmatic behavior observed in this study suggest that the following guidelines for contextual intervention may facilitate communication in end-stage Alzheimer's. Although most of these guidelines are derived from quantitative analysis of the data, Guidelines 1 and 2 and Guidelines 13 and 14 are based on techniques found effective by interlocutors during the process of data collection.

1. Preface attempts to communicate with attention-arousing signals, such as touch or addressing the patient by name.
2. Give the patient sufficient start-up time for joining conversations.
3. Allow long latencies for responding.
4. If the patient does not respond, repeat or rephrase message.
5. When the patient's message is unclear, request clarification.
6. If the patient does not provide clarification, state what you understood; then ask for confirmation.
7. Make use of contextual cues in interpreting the patient's message.
8. Supplement verbal message with physical contextual cues when addressing the patient.
9. Replace open-ended questions with questions that allow for yes–no responses, or provide two choices.
10. Continue use of social lubricants even when other communication seems ineffective.
11. Expect fluctuation in communicative performance within the individual patient.
12. Expect variation in communicative skills from patient to patient.
13. Provide frequent opportunities for communication, but do not expect the patient to initiate conversation.
14. Be prepared to make several attempts to engage the patient in conversation.

We maintain that it is worthwhile attempting to communicate with end-stage Alzheimer's patients even if they initially withdraw or resist communication. For example, Subject I.E., one of the least responsive of the 10 subjects, remarked at the end of a conversation, "I'm glad you talked to me." This suggests that a desire to communicate may be hidden by withdrawal or reduced initiative of communication.

Implications for Future Research

Although this study has identified several of the specific pragmatic strengths and weaknesses as well as general patterns of communication found in end-stage Alzheimer's disease, other important aspects remain largely unexplored. One area that warrants further investigation is the range of communicative intentions or functions within the repertoire of this population. In this study more information was obtained about the protocol of discourse than about the functions of discourse. A clearer picture of the latter might be gained by analyzing a larger conversational sample or by modifying certain aspects of the methodology. Davis and Wilcox (1985), for instance, reviewed several studies in which methods such as elicited conversation and structured tasks were used effectively in studying specific communicative functions.

Another important yet relatively unexplored area concerns the receptive pragmatic skills of individuals with end-stage Alzheimer's disease. Whereas this study placed more emphasis on production of pragmatic behaviors, important information remains to be gleaned from exploring those qualities of the interlocutor's pragmatic behavior that may contribute to successful communication. There are a number of reports concerning the ameliorative effects of certain nonverbal aspects of communication. Whitaker (1976) reported that eye contact facilitated comprehension in the subject described in her study of late mid-stage dementia. Langland and Panicucci (1982) reported that verbal communication accompanied by touch was more effective than verbal communication alone in communicating with "elderly, confused" patients. Bartol (1979) described several features of nonverbal behavior that were related to communicative success in advanced Alzheimer's disease. These included eye contact, facial expression, touch, gestures, and other nonrepresentational arm and hand movements. In addition, Bartol (1979) observed that her subjects were highly sensitive to such paralinguistic aspects of communication as rate, loudness, pitch, and intonation, especially as these are used to convey affect.

Data from the current study suggest that the population of individuals with advanced Alzheimer's disease may contain subgroups with distinct patterns of pragmatic behaviors. Further research with larger groups of subjects, in addition to improving external validity of the current findings, might identify these subgroups more accurately and account for their existence on the basis of biographical information or neuropathological differences. Identification of subgroups may provide a basis for differential methods of treatment.

This study did not examine differences in interaction between patients and familiar versus unfamiliar partners. If patients, even at this advanced stage, are more responsive to familiar partners, this information might be used to improve quality of care. Systematic exploration is needed, also, to determine whether other modifications in the communicative context, such as those proposed in the previous subsection, do indeed facilitate communication in end-stage Alzheimer's disease.

Finally, because this study was necessarily exploratory and the results preliminary, replication of this work with improved reliability in methodology would strengthen the validity of the results.

APPENDIX: GLOSSARY OF PRAGMATIC PARAMETERS

Control of topic: This parameter served to examine whether each utterance had a discernible theme and how that theme was introduced, maintained, or concluded during the discourse. A "discernible" topic was not necessarily discernible on the basis of a single utterance or turn, but was often recognizable from the linguistic or nonlinguistic context. Among the issues considered within this category were: (a) whether the theme of an utterance was introduced by the subject or by the conversational partner; (b) whether, when a new theme was introduced, the listener was adequately prepared for it, and whether the previous theme had been concluded appropriately; and (c) whether, when the subject continued a theme introduced earlier in the discourse, it was a theme initially raised by the subject him or herself or by the interlocutor.

Turns: A subject's turn was defined operationally as one of the following: (a) one or more consecutive utterances, gestures, actions, or communicative facial expressions by a subject including an unfilled pause of no more than 5 seconds; or (b) an interval of 3 to 30 seconds between two of the interlocutor's utterances during which the subject is expected (by the partner) to communicate but does not.

The two dimensions of turns examined were length and latency. In order for length to be judged appropriate, a subject's communicative act needed to be long enough to satisfy the discourse demands at that point in the conversation. For example, if an explanation were required, a yes or no response would be judged too short to fit the discourse requirements. On the other hand, a turn would be considered too long if it exceeded the length appropriate for the discourse demands.

Latency of turns concerns the interval between the subject's initiation of communication and the end of the interlocutor's previous turn. Garvey and Berninger (1981) reported that, in English, a latency of longer than 1 second signals a speaker's intention to forfeit the floor. In this study, a latency of over 3 seconds was considered inappropriately long. On the other hand, a negative latency, such as an interruption or press of speech, was also judged inappropriate.

Feedback to conversational partner: Speakers of American English usually signal to a conversational partner that her or his message has or has not been understood and/or that one agrees with, disagrees with, or neutrally accepts the message. Feedback can be verbal (e.g., "yea," "um-hum," or "really?") or nonverbal (e.g., a head nod or a puzzled facial expression). In the current study, any signals of this type were judged appropriate.

Presuppositions: According to Roth and Spekman (1984), making appropriate presuppositions requires correct assessment of shared information based on: (a) shared aspects of the physical setting; (b) general knowledge of the speaking situation or of the speaker's past experiences; or (c) monitoring of the preceding discourse. In the current study, the following behaviors were monitored for correct assessment of shared information: (a) informativeness, (b) deixis, (c) marking new and old information, (d) cohesion, and (e) appreciation of physical context.

Requesting repairs: For this pragmatic category, discourse was monitored to determine whether subjects asked the interlocutor to clarify a previous message when needed. Appropriate requests for repair could include verbal requests, such as "What did you say?" or "What do you mean?" or nonverbal requests, such as a facial expression conveying puzzlement.

Making repairs: Discourse samples were monitored to determine whether subjects attempted to clarify messages when the interlocutor indicated that she or he had not understood. Each attempt to make a repair was classified according to which of the following strategies was used: repetition, stress change, volume change, lexical change, phonological change, confirmation, specification, elaboration, demonstration, or other.

Social lubricants: This category includes boundary markers indicating openings ("Hi," "Come in") and closings ("Bye," "Come back again") as well as other social routines and politeness markers (such as, "Thanks," "Sorry," "Please").

Directives: According to Hutchinson and Jensen (1980), directives are communicative acts that serve to "get the listener(s) to do something" (p. 63). Questions, requests, and commands are included in this category. Specific directive behaviors examined in this study are: (a) expressions of personal need or desire; (b) imperatives; (c) warnings; (d) hints; (e) requests for objects, information, action, clarification, confirmation, or attention; and (f) transferring objects.

Responses to directives: This parameter concerns any signal that might be given to the conversational partner that a directive has or has not been understood. The signal may consist of a verbal response, such as, "okay," "no," or "later," or provision of the information requested. A nonverbal response, such as carrying out the directive, would also serve as an appropriate response.

Comments and representatives: This parameter includes statements of facts, rules, attitudes, judgments, beliefs about another's internal states, and explanations. According to Hutchinson and Jensen (1980), "Representatives convey the belief that some proposition is true" and usually "take the form of assertions or hypotheses" (p. 63). This parameter also includes descriptions of state or condition and descriptions of on-going, past, and future activities.

Acknowledging comments: This category concerns any signal, verbal or nonverbal, that a comment (assertion or representative) has or has not been understood. Acknowledgment may be positive (signaling agreement or approval) or neutral or negative (signaling disagreement or disapproval).

Expressives: This parameter concerns statements about the speaker's internal state, including expression of emotions, sensations, and mental events. A common form of expressives is a statement about how one feels.

Commissives: This parameter includes promises, pledges, vows, and guarantees. As defined by Hutchinson and Jensen (1980), "Commissives commit the speaker to some future course of action" (p. 63).

REFERENCES

Albert, M. L. (1980). Language in normal and dementing elderly. In L. Obler & M. Albert (Eds.), *Language and communication in the elderly* (pp. 145–150). Lexington, MA: D.C. Heath.

Bartol, M. (1979). Nonverbal communication in patients with Alzheimer's disease. *Journal of Gerontological Nursing, 54*, 21–31.

Bayles, K., Kaszniak, A., & Tomoeda, C. (1987). *Communication and cognition in normal aging and dementia.* San Diego: College Hill Press.

Bayles, K., Tomoeda, C., & Caffrey, J. (1982). Language and dementia producing diseases. *Communicative Disorders, 7,* 131–146.

Cairns, R. B., & Green, J. A. (1979). How to assess personality and social patterns: Observations or ratings? In R. B. Cairns (Ed.), *The analysis of social interactions: Methods, issues, and illustrations* (pp. 209–226). Hillsdale, NJ: Lawrence Erlbaum Associates.

Coulthard, M. (1977). *An introduction to discourse analysis.* London: Longman.

Davis, G. A., & Wilcox, M. J. (1985). *Adult aphasia rehabilitation: Applied pragmatics.* San Diego: College Hill Press.

de Ajuriaguerra, J., & Tissot, R. (1975). Some aspects of language in various forms of senile dementia (comparisons with language in childhood). In E. Lenneberg & E. Lenneberg (Eds.), *Foundations of language development: A multidisciplinary approach* (Vol. 1, pp. 323–339). New York: Academic Press.

Duchan, J. (1984). Language assessment: The pragmatics revolution. In R. C. Naremore (Ed.), *Language sciences: Recent advances* (pp. 147–180). San Diego: College Hill Press.

Garvey, C., & Berninger, G. (1981). Timing and turn-taking in children's conversations. *Discourse Processes, 4,* 27–57.

Hachinski, V. C. (1983). Differential diagnosis of Alzheimer's dementia: Multi-infarct dementia. In B. Reisberg (Ed.), *Alzheimer's disease: The standard reference* (pp. 188–192). New York: The Free Press.

Holland, A. L. (1982). Observing functional communication of aphasic adults. *Journal of Speech and Hearing Disorders, 47,* 50–56.

Hutchinson, J., & Jensen, M. (1980). A pragmatic evaluation of discourse communication in normal and senile elderly in a nursing home. In L. Obler & M. Albert (Eds.), *Language and communication in the elderly* (pp. 59–73). Lexington, MA: D.C. Heath.

Langland, R. M., & Panicucci, C. L. (1982). Tactile communication in elderly, confused clients. *Journal of Gerontological Nursing, 8,* 152–155.

Lubinski, R. (1981). Language and aging: An environmental approach to intervention. *Topics in Language Disorders, 2,* 89–97.

Manheim, H. L., & Simon, B. A. (1977). *Sociological research: Philosophy and methods.* Homewood, IL: The Dorsey Press.

Mahoney, F. I., & Barthel, D. W. (1965). Functional evaluation: The Barthel Index. *Maryland State Medical Journal, 14,* 61–65.

Mattis, S. (1976). Dementia Rating Scale. In R. Bellack & B. Karasu (Eds.), *Geriatric psychiatry* (pp. 97–104). New York: Raven Press.

McKhann, G., Drachman, D., Folstein, M, Katzman, R., Price, D., & Stadlan, E. M. (1984). Clinical diagnosis of Alzheimer's disease: Report of the NINCDS-ADRDA Work Group under the auspices of the Department of Health and Human Services Task Force on Alzheimer's Disease. *Neurology, 34,* 939–944.

Milligan, G. W. (1980). An examination of the effect of six types of error perturbation on 15 clustering algorithms. *Psychometrika, 45,* 325–342.

Obler, L. K. (1981). Review of *Le langage des déments. Brain and Language, 12,* 375–386.

Obler, L. K., & Albert, M. L. (1984). Language in aging. In M. L. Albert (Ed.), *Clinical neurology of aging* (pp. 245–253). New York: Oxford University Press.

Ostuni, E., & Santo Pietro, M. J. (1987). *Getting through: Communicating when someone you care for has Alzheimer's disease.* Plainsboro, NJ: The Speech Bin.

Parke, R. D. (1979). Interactional designs. In R. B. Cairns (Ed.), *The analysis of social interactions: Methods, issues and illustrations* (pp. 15–36). Hillsdale, NJ: Lawrence Erlbaum Associates.

Prutting, C. A., & Kirchner D. (1983). Applied pragmatics. In T. Gallagher & C. A. Prutting (Eds.), *Pragmatic assessment and intervention issues in language* (pp. 29–64). San Diego: College Hill Press.

Roth, F., & Spekman, N. (1984). Assessing the pragmatic abilities of children: Part 1. Organizational framework and assessment parameters. *Journal of Speech and Hearing Disorders, 47*, 2–11.

Schwartz, M. F., Marin, O. S. M., & Saffran, E. M. (1979). Dissociations of language function in dementia: A case study. *Brain and Language, 7*, 277–306.

Tonkovich, J. (1984). Dementia. *Communicative Disorders, 9*, 184–188.

Whitaker, H. A. (1976). A case of isolation of the language function. In H. Whitaker & H. A. Whitaker (Eds.), *Studies in neurolinguistics* (Vol. 2, pp. 1–58). New York: Academic Press.

Yarrow, M. R., & Waxler, C. Z. (1979). Observing interaction: A confrontation with methodology. In R. B. Cairns (Ed.), *The analysis of social interactions: Methods, issues, and illustrations* (pp. 37–66). Hillsdale, NJ: Lawrence Erlbaum Associates.

Author Index

Subject Index

U

V

W

For Product Safety Concerns and Information please contact our EU representative GPSR@taylorandfrancis.com
Taylor & Francis Verlag GmbH, Kaufingerstraße 24, 80331 München, Germany

www.ingramcontent.com/pod-product-compliance
Ingram Content Group UK Ltd.
Pitfield, Milton Keynes, MK11 3LW, UK
UKHW022001180926
475701UK00003B/134
9781138876408